Brain, Stroke and Kidney

Contributions to Nephrology

Vol. 179

Series Editor

Claudio Ronco Vicenza

Brain, Stroke and Kidney

Volume Editor

Kazunori Toyoda Osaka

21 figures and 20 tables, 2013

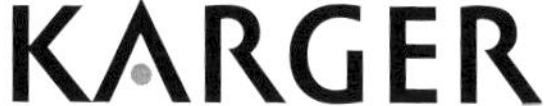

Basel · Freiburg · Paris · London · New York · New Delhi · Bangkok · Beijing · Tokyo · Kuala Lumpur · Singapore · Sydney

Contributions to Nephrology
(Founded 1975 by Geoffrey M. Berlyne)

Kazunori Toyoda
Department of Cerebrovascular Medicine
National Cerebral and Cardiovascular Center
5-7-1 Fujishirodai, Suita
Osaka, 565-8565
Japan

Library of Congress Cataloging-in-Publication Data

Brain, stroke, and kidney / volume editor, Kazunori Toyoda.
p. ; cm. -- (Contributions to nephrology, ISSN 0302-5144 ; v. 179)
Includes bibliographical references and indexes.
ISBN 978-3-318-02351-0 (alk. paper) -- ISBN 978-3-318-02352-7 (e-ISBN)
I. Toyoda, Kazunori (Physician) II. Series: Contributions to nephrology ; v. 179. 0302-5144
[DNLM: 1. Stroke--physiopathology. 2. Kidney Diseases--complications. 3. Stroke--prevention & control. 4. Stroke--therapy. W1 CO778UN v.179 2013 / WL 356]
RC388.5
616.8'1--dc23
2013008815

Bibliographic Indices. This publication is listed in bibliographic services, including Current Contents® and Index Medicus.

www.karger.com
Printed in Germany on acid-free and non-aging paper (ISO 9706) by Bosch Druck, Ergolding
ISSN 0302–5144
e-ISSN 1662–2782
ISBN 978–3–318–02351–0
e-ISBN 978–3–318–02352–7

Contents

Management for Stroke in Kidney Disease

Toyoda K (ed): Brain, Stroke and Kidney.
Contrib Nephrol. Basel, Karger, 2013, vol 179, pp 1–6 (DOI: 10.1159/000346944)

Cerebrorenal Interaction and Stroke

Kazunori Toyoda

Department of Cerebrovascular Medicine, National Cerebral and Cardiovascular Center, Suita, Osaka, Japan

Abstract

Beyond the original meaning of chronic kidney disease (CKD) as high-risk state for future dialysis, CKD is now known as an established risk factor for cardiovascular diseases. Stroke is a major player of cardiovascular disease and has deep two-way relationships with CKD. CKD is an evident risk factor for stroke. Meta-analyses of cohort studies and trials indicate that proteinuria/albuminuria increases the risk of stroke by 71–92%, and reduced glomerular filtration rate increases the risk by 43%. In addition, CKD has a strong relationship with subclinical brain damage including white matter changes, microbleeds, cognitive impairment, and carotid atherosclerosis. CKD is prevalent in acute stroke patients; patients with estimated glomerular filtration rate <60 ml/min/1.73 m^2 or proteinuria amounted to 46% of total ischemic stroke patients and 39% of total intracerebral hemorrhage patients in our institute. Acute and chronic management of stroke are influenced by CKD. Therapeutic effects of several antithrombotic and thrombolytic agents, including recently-developed novel oral anticoagulants, are affected by renal function. Moreover, reduced glomerular filtration rate is independently associated with increased 1- and 10-year mortalities in the end. Stroke also has deep relationships with end-stage kidney disease. Stroke occurs much more commonly in dialysis patients than general population or CKD patients without need for dialysis. The triggers of ischemic and hemorrhagic stroke in patients with end-stage kidney disease include special characteristics unique to dialysis, such as drastic hemodynamic change, dialysate and anticoagulants, and vascular calcification. As cohorts of dialysis patients become older, more hypertensive, and more diabetic than before, stroke become more prevalent and more serious events in dialysis clinics. Now, clinicians should have much interest in the association between CKD and cerebrovascular diseases, so-called the cerebro-renal interaction.

More than ten years have passed since the National Kidney Foundation in the United States first advocated the concept of chronic kidney disease (CKD) [1], and it is now seen as a major public health problem. According to the 2002 ver-

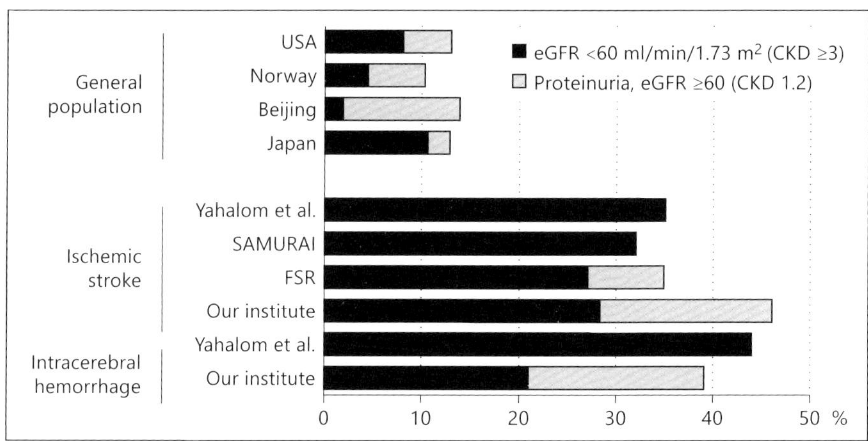

Fig. 1. The prevalence of eGFR <60 ml/min/1.73 m^2 or proteinuria in both the general population and stroke patients. Cited from refs. 2–5 and 12–14. Note that both eGFR and proteinuria in stroke patients were measured during the acute stage of stroke, and thereby might have been affected by stroke damage.

sion of the guideline, the prevalence estimates of CKD in the United States (1999–2004) were as follows [1]: 1.8% (95% CI 1.4–2.3%) for stage 1 (estimated glomerular filtration rate (eGFR) >90 ml/min/1.73 m^2 and albuminuria); 3.2% (95% CI 2.6–3.9%) for stage 2 (GFR 60–89 ml/min/1.73 m^2 and albuminuria); 7.7% (95% CI 7.0–8.4%) for stage 3 (GFR 30–59 ml/min/1.73 m^2), and 0.35% (0.25–0.45%) for stage 4 (GFR 15–29 ml/min/1.73 m^2) [2]. Estimates were 2.7 ± 0.3, 3.2 ± 0.4, 4.2 ± 0.1, and 0.2 ± 0.01%, respectively, in Norway (1995–1997) [3]; 7.4% (95% CI 6.9–7.8%), 4.7% (4.4–5.1%), 1.8% (1.5–2.0%), and none, respectively, in Beijing [4], and 0.6, 1.7, 10.4, and 0.2% (including CKD stage 5 without dialysis), respectively, in Japan (2005) [5] (fig. 1). Thus, more than one tenth of the general population worldwide is estimated to have CKD, and its prevalence increases dramatically with age.

Beyond the original meaning of CKD as a high-risk state for future dialysis, CKD is now known to be an established risk factor for cardiovascular diseases. This message was clarified by the Kaiser Permanente Renal Registry involving more than one million adults [6]. An independent, graded association was observed between a reduced eGFR and the risk of death and cardiovascular events including stroke. Since then, many studies have proven the positive association of CKD with risk and outcomes of cardiovascular disease. The reason for the positive association is partly the high prevalence of traditional cardiovascular risk factors in CKD patients. In addition, nontraditional risk factors, including endothelial dysfunction, maladaptive arterial remodeling, homocysteinemia, coagulation disorders, impaired endothelial release of tissue plasminogen activator (t-PA), extravascular coagulation, anemia, and higher levels of inflammatory cytokines and oxidative stress, seem to increase the risk of cardiovascular disease. In 2008, a consensus conference on cardiorenal syndromes was held to identify and classify dysfunction of the heart and kidneys whereby acute or chronic dysfunction in one organ induces acute or chronic dysfunction in the other organ [7]. Now, cardiologists cannot overlook CKD.

Stroke is a major player in cardiovascular disease and it has strong two-way relationships with CKD. Nevertheless, clinicians are often more indifferent to the association between CKD and cerebrovascular diseases, the so-called cerebrorenal interaction, than the cardiorenal interaction [8]. For example, cerebrovascular disease was rarely discussed in the lengthy *Contributions to Nephrology* series. This may be due to the fact that both renal and cerebral pathophysiologies are quite difficult for nonexperts to grasp and fully understand. Therefore, we have prepared this volume entitled 'Brain, stroke, and kidney'.

Now, let us think about the cerebrorenal interaction, particularly with respect to stroke. First, the glomerular afferent arterioles of the juxtamedullary nephrons and the cerebral perforating arteries share an anatomical feature. These small, short vessels directly arise from large high-pressure arteries, and are thus exposed to high pressure. They have to maintain a strong vascular tone in order to provide a large pressure gradient over a short distance [9]. Severe hypertensive vascular damage occurs first in such strain vessels. Since albuminuria reflects glomerular damage distal to the juxtamedullary afferent arterioles, albuminuria may also be an early sign of damage to the cerebral perforating arteries.

Second, CKD is an evident risk factor for stroke. Meta-analyses of both cohort studies and trials indicate that proteinuria/albuminuria increases the risk of stroke by 71–92% [10], and reduced eGFR (<60 ml/min/1.73 m^2) increases the risk by 43% [11]. In addition, CKD has a strong relationship with subclinical brain damage, including white matter changes, microbleeds, cognitive impairment, and carotid atherosclerosis. Of these, cognitive impairment and dementia are becoming as serious a burden as stroke worldwide.

Third, CKD is prevalent in acute stroke patients. Patients with eGFR <60 ml/min/1.73 m^2 based on the creatinine level during acute stroke accounted for 35% of total ischemic stroke patients and 44% of total intracerebral hemorrhage (ICH) patients in an Israeli hospital [12], and 32% of total patients receiving intravenous recombinant t-PA from the Stroke Acute Management with Urgent Risk-factor Assessment and Improvement (SAMURAI) rt-PA Registry in Japan

[13]. Patients with eGFR <60 ml/min/1.73 m^2 or proteinuria accounted for 46% of total ischemic stroke patients and 39% of total ICH patients in our institute and 34.9% of total ischemic stroke patients in the Fukuoka Stroke Registry [14] (fig. 1).

Fourth, acute and chronic stroke management strategies are influenced by CKD. A good example of this is the recently developed novel oral anticoagulants. Atrial fibrillation is a major risk factor for initial and recurrent stroke. To judge the indications and dosage of dabigatran and factor Xa inhibitors for stroke patients having atrial fibrillation, many neurologists are now familiar with the Cockcroft-Gault equations. Therapeutic effects of other antithrombotic and thrombolytic agents also seem to be affected by renal function. For example, in our multicenter SAMURAI rt-PA Registry [13], reduced eGFR was associated with early symptomatic ICH, mortality, and a modified Rankin scale score ≥4 at 3 months after intravenous thrombolysis in ischemic stroke patients.

Fifth, reduced eGFR is independently associated with increased 1- and 10-year mortalities [12, 15]. Two groups reported that proteinuria, but not a reduced eGFR, was associated with a poor functional outcome after ischemic stroke [14, 16]. Thus, the kidneys cannot be ignored by stroke neurologists.

Stroke also has strong relationships with end-stage kidney disease (ESKD). Stroke and other cardiovascular diseases occur much more commonly in dialysis patients than in the general population or in CKD patients who do not require dialysis [17, 18]. The triggers for ischemic and hemorrhagic strokes in ESKD patients include traditional cardiovascular risk factors, CKD-related nontraditional risk factors, and special characteristics unique to dialysis, such as drastic hemodynamic change, dialysate, anticoagulants, and vascular calcification. As cohorts of dialysis patients become older, more hypertensive, and more diabetic than before, strokes become more prevalent and more serious events in dialysis clinics. Strokes in ESKD patients pose problems, such as the contraindication to some pharmacotherapy (like dabigatran) and the difficulty of continuing dialysis under good conditions when severe neurological deficits remain. Though thrombolysis is not contraindicated for ESKD patients, even thrombolysis experts often have had limited experience with this therapy for ESKD patients [19].

In this volume, clinical and epidemiological specialists on 'Brain, stroke and kidney' present superb reviews for clinicians. I hope that you, the reader, enjoy this collection and that it promotes both further understanding and multidisciplinary collaboration between nephrologists and neurologists.

Acknowledgements

Our series of studies on the present theme was supported in part by a Grant-in-Aid for Scientific Research (23591288) from the Japan Society for the Promotion of Science, a Grant-in-Aid (H23-Junkanki-Ippan-010) from the Ministry of Health, Labor and Welfare, Japan, and an Intramural Research Fund (H23-4-3) for Cardiovascular Diseases of the National Cerebral and Cardiovascular Center.

References

1 National Kidney Foundation: K/DOQI clinical practice guidelines for chronic kidney disease: evaluation, classification, and stratification. Am J Kidney Dis 2002; 39:S1–S266.
2 Hallan SI, Coresh J, Astor BC, Asberg A, Powe NR, Romundstad S, Hallan HA, Lydersen S, Holmen J: International comparison of the relationship of chronic kidney disease prevalence and ESRD risk. J Am Soc Nephrol 2006;17:2275–2284.
3 Longenecker JC, Coresh J, Powe NR, Levey AS, Fink NE, Martin A, Klag MJ: Traditional cardiovascular disease risk factors in dialysis patients compared with the general population: the CHOICE Study. J Am Soc Nephrol 2002;13:1918–1927.
4 Zhang L, Zhang P, Wang F, Zuo L, Zhou Y, Shi Y, Li G, Jiao S, Liu Z, Liang W, Wang H: Prevalence and factors associated with CKD: a population study from Beijing. Am J Kidney Dis 2008;51:373–384.
5 Imai E, Horio M, Watanabe T, Iseki K, Yamagata K, Hara S, Ura N, Kiyohara Y, Moriyama T, Ando Y, Fujimoto S, Konta T, Yokoyama H, Makino H, Hishida A, Matsuo S: Prevalence of chronic kidney disease in the Japanese general population. Clin Exp Nephrol 2009;13:621–630.
6 Go AS, Chertow GM, Fan D, McCulloch CE, Hsu CY: Chronic kidney disease and the risks of death, cardiovascular events, and hospitalization. N Engl J Med 2004;351:1296–1305.
7 Ronco C, McCullough P, Anker SD, Anand I, Aspromonte N, Bagshaw SM, Bellomo R, Berl T, Bobek I, Cruz DN, Daliento L, Davenport A, Haapio M, Hillege H, House AA, Katz N, Maisel A, Mankad S, Zanco P, Mebazaa A, Palazzuoli A, Ronco F, Shaw A, Sheinfeld G, Soni S, Vescovo G, Zamperetti N, Ponikowski P, Acute Dialysis Quality Initiative (ADQI) Consensus Group: Cardio-renal syndromes: report from the consensus conference of the acute dialysis quality initiative. Eur Heart J 2010;31:703–711.
8 Toyoda K: The cerebro-renal interaction in stroke neurology. Neurology 2012;78:1898–1899.
9 Ito S, Nagasawa T, Abe M, Mori T: Strain vessel hypothesis: a viewpoint for linkage of albuminuria and cerebro-cardiovascular risk. Hypertens Res 2009;32:115–121.
10 Lee M, Saver JL, Chang KH, Liao HW, Chang SC, Ovbiagele B: Low glomerular filtration rate and risk of stroke: meta-analysis. BMJ 2010;341:c4249.
11 Lee M, Saver JL, Chang KH, Liao HW, Chang SC, Ovbiagele B: Impact of microalbuminuria on incident stroke: a meta-analysis. Stroke 2010;41:2625–2631.
12 Yahalom G, Schwartz R, Schwammenthal Y, Merzeliak O, Toashi M, Orion D, Sela BA, Tanne D: Chronic kidney disease and clinical outcome in patients with acute stroke. Stroke 2009;40:1296–1303.
13 Naganuma M, Koga M, Shiokawa Y, Nakagawara J, Furui E, Kimura K, Yamagami H, Okada Y, Hasegawa Y, Kario K, Okuda S, Nishiyama K, Minematsu K, Toyoda K: Reduced estimated glomerular filtration rate is associated with stroke outcomes after intravenous rt-PA: the Stroke Acute Management with Urgent Risk-factor Assessment and Improvement (SAMURAI) rt-PA Registry. Cerebrovasc Dis 2011;31: 123–129.
14 Kumai Y, Kamouchi M, Hata J, Ago T, Kitayama J, Nakane H, Sugimori H, Kitazono T: Proteinuria and clinical outcomes after ischemic stroke. Neurology 2012;78:1909–1915

15 Tsagalis G, Akrivos T, Alevizaki M, Manios E, Stamatellopoulos K, Laggouranis A, Vemmos KN: Renal dysfunction in acute stroke: an independent predictor of long-term all combined vascular events and overall mortality. Nephrol Dial Transplant 2009;24:194–200.
16 Ovbiagele B, Sanossian N, Liebeskind DS, Kim D, Ali LK, Pineda S, Saver JL: Indices of kidney dysfunction and discharge outcomes in hospitalized stroke patients without known renal disease. Cerebrovasc Dis 2009; 28:582–588.
17 Toyoda K, Fujii K, Ando T, Kumai Y, Ibayashi S, Iida M: Incidence, etiology, and outcome of stroke in patients on continuous ambulatory peritoneal dialysis. Cerebrovasc Dis 2004;17:98–105.
18 Toyoda K, Fujii K, Fujimi S, Kumai Y, Tsuchimochi H, Ibayashi S, Iida M: Stroke in patients on maintenance hemodialysis: a 22-year single-center study. Am J Kidney Dis 2005;45:1058–1066.
19 Palacio S, Gonzales NR, Sangha NS, Birnbaum LA, Hart RG: Thrombolysis for acute stroke in hemodialysis: international survey of expert opinion. Clin J Am Soc Nephrol 2011;6:1089–1093.

Kazunori Toyoda, MD
Department of Cerebrovascular Medicine
National Cerebral and Cardiovascular Center
5-7-1 Fujishiro-dai, Suita, Osaka 565-8565 (Japan)
E-Mail toyoda@hsp.ncvc.go.jp

Toyoda K (ed): Brain, Stroke and Kidney.
Contrib Nephrol. Basel, Karger, 2013, vol 179, pp 7–14 (DOI: 10.1159/000346717)

Inhibition of the Renin-Angiotensin-Aldosterone System for Cerebrorenal Protection

H.J. Lambers Heerspink

Department of Clinical Pharmacology, University Medical Center Groningen, University of Groningen, Groningen, The Netherlands

Abstract

Blood pressure is a strong risk factor for ischemic and atherosclerotic events such as stroke. Blood pressure is often elevated in patients with chronic kidney disease. Consequently, chronic kidney disease patients are at high risk of developing cardiovascular and cerebrovascular damage. Blood pressure reduction by means of inhibiting the renin-angiotensin-aldosterone system (RAAS) reduces the risk of stroke. There is evidence available in the primary and secondary prevention of stroke that RAAS blockade exerts cerebrovascular protective effects independent of blood pressure lowering. This chapter discusses the role of RAAS blockade for the prevention and treatment of stroke in chronic kidney disease. The role of dual RAAS blockade will be reviewed and alternative strategies to enhance the effects of angiotensin-converting enzyme inhibitors and angiotensin receptor blockers will be provided.

Patients with chronic kidney disease (CKD) face a high risk of end-stage renal disease and cardiovascular disease including stroke. Hypertension is common in CKD and affects 50–75% of all individuals [1]. Disturbed arterial blood pressure has been clearly established as a risk factor for stroke and even moderate increases in arterial blood pressure provoke cerebrovascular damage. Worldwide stroke accounts for almost one-third of all cardiovascular deaths. In light of the ageing population, industrialization of third-world countries, and increase in the prevalence of CKD, it is expected that the prevalence and economic burden of stroke increases.

Numerous studies have documented a continuous linear association between blood pressure and the presence of cerebrovascular disease. In CKD, epidemiological data show a stronger association between blood pressure and stroke as compared to individuals without CKD, at least in women [2]. In addition, it is well established that any form of blood pressure-lowering therapy decreases the risk of stroke. Results from meta-analyses indicate that for every 4 mm Hg blood pressure reduction the risk of stroke decreases by approximately 20% [3]. Next to blood pressure there are many other risk factors that increase cerebrovascular damage. Increased renin-angiotensin-aldosterone system (RAAS) activity, for example, causes endothelial dysfunction, chronic inflammation, and increases albuminuria. Hence, increased RAAS-activity is an important contributor of cerebrovascular damage in humans.

Historically, it was thought that the RAAS consists of a number of circulating hormones mediating vasoconstriction, glomerular filtration pressure, and aldosterone excretion. However, during recent years it has become increasingly apparent that the RAAS has a broad diversity of (patho)physiological effects including modulation of inflammation and regulation of cell growth and differentiation [4, 5]. Since the kidney is both the endocrine organ and target organ of the RAAS, the deleterious effects of angiotensin II, the primary mediator of the RAAS, are profoundly apparent in the kidney. Indeed, continued activation of the RAAS constricts renal arterioles leading to increased peripheral and renal resistance and triggers pro-inflammatory and profibrotic processes in the kidney contributing to progressive renal function loss [6, 7]. With respect to the cerebrovascular system, it has long been recognized that an independent regulated RAAS exists in the brain which thus acts independent of the circulating RAAS [8]. In the brain, increased angiotensin II activity affects cerebrovascular autoregulation and causes inflammation via activation of the AT1 receptor. The brain RAAS may also exert neuronal regeneration via activation of the AT2 receptor. The AT2 receptor is distributed mostly in the brain, vasculature, and myocardium and thus counterbalances the activity of the AT1 receptor. Indeed, genetically deleted mice those the AT1 receptor had decreased ischemic injury whereas it was increased in AT2 receptor-deficient mice [9, 10]. Thus, the balance between both receptor subtypes determines the ultimate outcome.

The importance of the RAAS in renal and cerebrovascular disease has received further recognition by the proven clinical benefits of agents intervening in the RAAS. The blood pressure-lowering effects of angiotensin converting enzyme inhibitors (ACEI) and angiotensin receptor blockers (ARBs) are well documented and they have been demonstrated to improve clinical outcomes in both renal and cerebrovascular disease [11, 12]. A number of randomized controlled trials have assessed the effects of ACEI or ARBs in preventing cerebrovascular events and some of them have specifically evaluated whether RAAS intervention within the first period after cerebrovascular damage prevented recurrent stroke. Unfortunately, none of these trials were specifically designed to assess the cerebrovascular or cardiovascular benefits of RAAS intervention in a broad range of CKD patients. Yet, in some trials, CKD patients were included and post hoc analyses of these trials have provided valuable insight into the effects of RAAS blockade in this population. An important finding that has been observed in a number of trials is that RAAS inhibition confers cardiovascular protection independent of its blood pressure-lowering effect.

Effect of RAAS Inhibition in the Primary Prevention of Stroke

The Heart Outcomes Protection Evaluation (HOPE) assessed the effect of ramipril on cardiovascular outcome in subjects at high risk of cardiovascular events. The study found that ramipril prevented the number of strokes by 32% despite a modest blood pressure difference between the placebo and active treatment arm [13]. A subsequent post hoc analysis showed that this reduction in risk of stroke was consistent in subjects with renal insufficiency or without renal insufficiency [14]. The initial interpretation of the trial suggested that the prevention of stroke could not be explained by the modest blood pressure difference between the two treatment arms. The 24-hour blood pressure data obtained in a selection of the HOPE participants, however, showed 10/4 mm Hg blood pressure reduction in the ramipril arm. This suggests that the observed blood pressure difference could account for the observed cardiovascular protective effect of ramipril.

In contrast to the HOPE results, the LIFE trial provided evidence that the protective effects of RAAS inhibition with the ARB losartan go beyond blood pressure reduction. The LIFE trial compared the effects of losartan versus the β-blocker atenolol in patients with essential hypertension and left-ventricular hypertrophy. The trial showed significant benefits with losartan in preventing cardiovascular events, which were driven by clear reductions in stroke [15]. Interestingly, the atenolol and losartan treatment regimen provided comparable reduction in blood pressure indicating blood pressure-independent benefits of losartan likely mediated by reductions in albuminuria. The benefits of RAAS inhibition, independent of blood pressure control, were also observed in the Kyoto Heart Study [16]. The Kyoto Heart Study randomly assigned 3,031 Japanese patients with uncontrolled hypertension to treatment with valsartan or placebo. The trial was prematurely discontinued after 3.3 years follow-up because of significant benefit with valsartan on stroke events despite similar blood pressure control in the valsartan and placebo treatment arm. Post-hoc analyses from this trial revealed that the reduction in cerebrovascular accidents with valsartan were similar in patients with and without CKD [17].

Effect of RAAS Inhibition in the Secondary Prevention of Stroke

After experiencing stroke, patients are at elevated risk to experience a recurrent stroke, and this often leads to premature death, even more so than after the first stroke. The available data indicate that patients high blood pressure is a major determinant of recurrent stroke. The largest trial of secondary stroke prevention that includes an ACEI is the PROGRESS trial. The PROGRESS trial showed that among patients with stroke or transient ischemic attack in the previous 8 months an ACEI (perindopril)-based regimen reduces blood pressure by 9.0/4.0 mm Hg and the risk of recurrent stroke by 28% [18]. In the PROGRESS trial, active treatment could consist of the ACEI perindopril or the combination of perindopril with the diuretic indapamide. Thus, the randomized study allocation in PROGRESS could either be single medication (perindopril) versus placebo or combination therapy (perindopril and indapamide) versus double placebo. Relative to placebo, combination therapy produced a 12.3/5.0 mm Hg blood pressure reduction and 43% relative risk reduction risk of recurrent stroke which was significantly greater than the 4.9/2.8 mm Hg blood pressure reduction and nonsignificant 5% risk reduction conferred by single therapy. A detailed post hoc analysis was conducted to assess whether the benefits of an ACEI-based regimen were equally present in CKD patients [19]. The results of this analysis showed indeed that the benefit of ACE inhibition to prevent recurrent stroke as well as major cardiovascular events were consistent in subjects with and without CKD. Importantly, in light of the higher risk of CKD subjects for cardiovascular and stroke events, the absolute risk reductions were markedly greater in CKD subjects. Consequently, much fewer patients needed to be treated to prevent one stroke event.

The difference in blood pressure throughout follow-up in the two treatment arms in PROGRESS precluded any inferences about blood pressure independent effects of the ACEI-based regimen. Therefore, the MOSES trial was designed with the aim to demonstrate that for the same level of blood pressure reduction the ARB eprosartan will be more effective in reducing cerebrovascular events than the calcium channel blocker nitrendipine in hypertensive stroke patients. During follow-up, similar blood pressure levels were achieved with eprosartan (138/81 mm Hg) and nitrendipine (136/80 mm Hg) [20]. Yet, treatment with eprosartan caused 25% fewer cerebrovascular events compared with nitrendipine providing additional support of blood pressure independent protective effects of RAAS inhibition.

The blood pressure reducing therapy in PROGRESS was initiated on average 8 months after stroke. The PRoFESS trial was designed to address the question whether earlier intervention would be beneficial. To this end, telmisartan was compared with placebo in 20,392 patients with prior ischemic stroke. The median interval between stroke and randomization in this study was 15 days and subsequent follow-up lasted for 2.5 years. During follow-up the blood pressure difference between both treatment arms was 3.8/2.0 mm Hg. The risk for recurrent stroke only decreased by 5% which was not statistically significant from placebo treatment ($p = 0.23$) [21]. How can we reconcile these outcomes in light of the PROGRESS and MOSES trials showing clear benefits of RAAS inhibition? The PRoFESS authors suggested that the lesser blood pressure reduction in PRoFESS compared to PROGRESS is a possible explanation. They note that the benefit in PROGRESS was seen in the combination perindopril-indapamide arm whereas the blood pressure reduction in the perindopril alone arm was of similar magnitude as in PRoFESS with a similar nonsignificant 5% relative risk reduction. In addition, modification of the underlying atherosclerotic process takes time and one can possibly not expect significant benefits in the early months of treatment. Indeed, a post hoc analysis showed that in PRoFESS no benefit was seen up to 6 months after randomization, but a small significant benefit was observed thereafter. The mean duration in PRoFESS was 2.5 years which might have been too short to detect a significant treatment effect.

Dual RAAS Inhibition in Prevention of Stroke

Various short-term studies on the blood pressure and albuminuria lowering effects of combination therapy with ACEIs and ARB fuelled the expectation that dual RAAS blockade would allow better long-term renal and cardiovascular/cerebrovascular outcome in CKD than single therapy. However, large-scale randomized controlled trials have reported contradictory results. In the ONTARGET trial, in patients with established cardiovascular disease of whom approximately one quarter had estimated glomerular filtration rates (eGFR) less than 60 ml/min, dual blockade with the ACEI ramipril and ARB telmisartan did not enhance cerebrovascular or renal protection [22]. The premature discontinuation of the ALTITUDE trial cast further doubt on the benefit of dual RAAS blockade in CKD. This trial studied the addition of aliskiren to losartan in patients with type 2 diabetes at high renal or cardiovascular risk [23]. The average eGFR in ALTITUDE was 51 ml/min/1.73 m^2 [24]. The safety monitoring board recommended early trial termination, based on lack of efficacy and higher rate of adverse events, particularly hyperkalemia and acute renal function loss. The final study data report a trend towards increased risk of stroke with the addition of aliskiren to losartan. Whether the lack of benefit with dual RAAS blockade is specific to the study populations, or the specific drug regimens in ONTARGET or ALTITUDE, is not yet established.

Dietary Sodium Restriction and RAAS Inhibition

Are other strategies apart from dual RAAS inhibition available to reduce the burden of stroke in CKD? A high salt intake causes a rise in blood pressure which in turn increases the risk of stroke. Apart from effects mediated through blood pressure, experimental data have shown that high salt intake may increase stroke risk directly [25]. An ecological study of the relation between urinary sodium excretion data and stroke mortality in Western Europe showed a significant positive correlation [26].

It has been known for over 20 years that dietary sodium restriction enhances the efficacy of RAAS blockade, in hypertension, in diabetic [27, 28], and in non-diabetic CKD [29]. Sodium restriction enhances the responses of both blood pressure and proteinuria to RAAS-blockade by a shift of the top of the dose response, so that a larger maximum effect can be obtained. The potentiation occurs with all available RAAS blocking agents, including ACEi [30], ARB [31], their combination [29], and renin inhibition [32]. Recent data in subjects with type 2 diabetes and nephropathy showed that the larger reduction in blood pressure and albuminuria during dietary sodium restriction and RAAS blockade translate in a larger reduction in the incidence of hard cardiovascular outcomes, including stroke [33]. These data suggest that optimization of sodium status has great potential to improve outcome in CKD, in particular considering the high dietary salt intake in CKD [34].

In summary, CKD is associated with considerable cardiovascular and cerebrovascular disease. Elevated blood pressure is a main determinant of cerebrovascular damage and blood pressure reduction reduces the risk of stroke. A growing number of studies show that blood pressure reduction obtained by RAAS blockade has an additive cerebrovascular protective effect. Combining multiple RAAS-inhibiting agents is not recommended and may even be harmful. In contrast, avoiding high dietary sodium intake against a background of RAAS blockade seems to be an effective strategy to further mitigate the burden of cardiovascular and cerebrovascular disease in patients with CKD.

References

1 K/DOQI clinical practice guidelines on hypertension and antihypertensive agents in chronic kidney disease. Am J Kidney Dis 2004;43(suppl 1):S1–S290.
2 Kokubo Y, Nakamura S, Okamura T, et al: Relationship between blood pressure category and incidence of stroke and myocardial infarction in an urban Japanese population with and without chronic kidney disease: the Suita Study. Stroke 2009;40:2674–2679.
3 Turnbull F: Effects of different blood-pressure-lowering regimens on major cardiovascular events: results of prospectively-designed overviews of randomised trials. Lancet 2003; 362:1527–1535.
4 Ruiz-Ortega M, Lorenzo O, Suzuki Y, Ruperez M, Egido J: Proinflammatory actions of angiotensins. Curr Opin Nephrol Hypertens 2001;10:321–329.
5 Suzuki Y, Ruiz-Ortega M, Gomez-Guerrero C, Tomino Y, Egido J: Angiotensin II, the immune system and renal diseases: another road for RAS? Nephrol Dial Transplant 2003; 18:1423–1426.
6 Remuzzi G, Bertani T: Pathophysiology of progressive nephropathies. N Engl J Med 1998;339:1448–1456.
7 Yoshioka T, Rennke HG, Salant DJ, Deen WM, Ichikawa I: Role of abnormally high transmural pressure in the permselectivity defect of glomerular capillary wall: a study in early passive Heymann nephritis. Circ Res 1987;61:531–538.
8 Unger T, Badoer E, Ganten D, Lang RE, Rettig R: Brain angiotensin: pathways and pharmacology. Circulation 1988;77:I40–I54.
9 Walther T, Olah L, Harms C, et al: Ischemic injury in experimental stroke depends on angiotensin II. FASEB J 2002;16:169–176.
10 Iwai M, Liu HW, Chen R, et al: Possible inhibition of focal cerebral ischemia by angiotensin II type 2 receptor stimulation. Circulation 2004;110:843–848.
11 Ruggenenti P, Perna A, Gherardi G, et al: Renoprotective properties of ACE-inhibition in non-diabetic nephropathies with non-nephrotic proteinuria. Lancet 1999;354:359–364.
12 Brenner BM, Cooper ME, de Zeeuw D, et al: Effects of losartan on renal and cardiovascular outcomes in patients with type 2 diabetes and nephropathy. N Engl J Med 2001;345:861–869.
13 Bosch J, Yusuf S, Pogue J, et al: Use of ramipril in preventing stroke: double blind randomised trial. BMJ 2002;324:699–702.
14 Mann JF, Gerstein HC, Pogue J, Bosch J, Yusuf S: Renal insufficiency as a predictor of cardiovascular outcomes and the impact of ramipril: the HOPE randomized trial. Ann Intern Med 2001;134:629–636.
15 Dahlof B, Devereux RB, Kjeldsen SE, et al: Cardiovascular morbidity and mortality in the Losartan Intervention For Endpoint reduction in hypertension study (LIFE): a randomised trial against atenolol. Lancet 2002; 359:995–1003.
16 Sawada T, Yamada H, Dahlof B, Matsubara H: Effects of valsartan on morbidity and mortality in uncontrolled hypertensive patients with high cardiovascular risks: KYOTO HEART Study. Eur Heart J 2009;30:2461–2469.
17 Amano K, Shiraishi J, Sawada T, Koide M, Yamada H, Matsubara H: Enhanced cardio-renal protective effects of valsartan in high-risk hypertensive patients with chronic kidney disease: a sub-analysis of KYOTO HEART Study. Int J Cardiol
18 Randomised trial of a perindopril-based blood-pressure-lowering regimen among 6,105 individuals with previous stroke or transient ischaemic attack. Lancet 2001;358: 1033–1041.
19 Perkovic V, Ninomiya T, Arima H, et al: Chronic kidney disease, cardiovascular events, and the effects of perindopril-based blood pressure lowering: data from the PROGRESS study. J Am Soc Nephrol 2007; 18:2766–2772.
20 Schrader J, Luders S, Kulschewski A, et al: Morbidity and mortality after stroke – eprosartan compared with nitrendipine for secondary prevention: principal results of a prospective randomized controlled study (MOSES). Stroke 2005;36:1218–1226.
21 Yusuf S, Diener HC, Sacco RL, et al: Telmisartan to prevent recurrent stroke and cardiovascular events. N Engl J Med 2008;359: 1225–1237.
22 Yusuf S, Teo KK, Pogue J, et al. Telmisartan, ramipril, or both in patients at high risk for vascular events. N Engl J Med 2008;358: 1547–1559.

23 Parving HH, Brenner BM, McMurray JJ, et al: Aliskiren Trial in Type 2 Diabetes Using Cardio-Renal Endpoints (ALTITUDE): rationale and study design. Nephrol Dial Transplant 2009;24:1663–1671.
24 Parving HH, Brenner BM, McMurray JJ, et al: Baseline characteristics in the Aliskiren Trial in Type 2 Diabetes Using Cardio-Renal Endpoints (ALTITUDE). J Renin Angiotensin Aldosterone Syst 2012;13:387–393.
25 Tobian L, Hanlon S: High sodium chloride diets injure arteries and raise mortality without changing blood pressure. Hypertension 1990;15:900–903.
26 Perry IJ, Beevers DG: Salt intake and stroke: a possible direct effect. J Hum Hypertens 1992; 6:23–25.
27 Houlihan CA, Allen TJ, Baxter AL, et al: A low-sodium diet potentiates the effects of losartan in type 2 diabetes. Diabetes Care 2002;25:663–671.
28 Ekinci EI, Thomas G, Thomas D, et al: Effects of salt supplementation on the albuminuric response to telmisartan with or without hydrochlorothiazide therapy in hypertensive patients with type 2 diabetes are modulated by habitual dietary salt intake. Diabetes Care 2009;32:1398–1403.
29 Slagman MC, Waanders F, Hemmelder MH, et al: Moderate dietary sodium restriction added to angiotensin converting enzyme inhibition compared with dual blockade in lowering proteinuria and blood pressure: randomised controlled trial. BMJ 2011; 343:d4366.
30 Heeg JE, de Jong PE, van der Hem GK, de Zeeuw D: Efficacy and variability of the antiproteinuric effect of ACE inhibition by lisinopril. Kidney Int 1989;36:272–279.
31 Vogt L, Waanders F, Boomsma F, de Zeeuw D, Navis G: Effects of dietary sodium and hydrochlorothiazide on the antiproteinuric efficacy of losartan. J Am Soc Nephrol 2008;19:999–1007.
32 Weir MR, Yadao AM, Purkayastha D, Charney AN: Effects of high- and low-sodium diets on ambulatory blood pressure in patients with hypertension receiving aliskiren. J Cardiovasc Pharmacol Ther 2010;15:356–363.
33 Heerspink HJ, Holtkamp FA, Parving HH, et al: Moderation of dietary sodium potentiates the renal and cardiovascular protective effects of angiotensin receptor blockers. Kidney Int 2012;82:330–337.
34 Krikken JA, Laverman GD, Navis G: Benefits of dietary sodium restriction in the management of chronic kidney disease. Curr Opin Nephrol Hypertens 2009;18:531–538.

H.J. Lambers Heerspink
Department of Clinical Pharmacology, University Medical Centre Groningen
University of Groningen, Ant Deusing laan 1
NL–9713 AV Groningen (The Netherlands)
E-Mail h.j.lambers.heerspink@umcg.nl

Toyoda K (ed): Brain, Stroke and Kidney.
Contrib Nephrol. Basel, Karger, 2013, vol 179, pp 15–23 (DOI: 10.1159/000346718)

Obesity and Heart Failure as a Mediator of the Cerebrorenal Interaction

Ankur Jindal · Adam Whaley-Connell · James R. Sowers

Department of Internal Medicine, University of Missouri, Columbia, Mo., USA

Abstract

The obesity epidemic is contributing substantially to the burden of cardiovascular disease including heart disease and congestive heart failure, in the United States and the rest of the world. Overnutrition as a driver of obesity, promotes alterations in fatty acid, lipid, and glucose metabolism that influence myocardial function and progression of heart failure from diastolic to systolic failure. The association of progressive heart failure and progressive chronic kidney disease is well documented and often referred to as the cardiorenal syndrome, as well as a prognosticator for cerebrovascular disease (e.g. stroke). Whether the relationship between obesity, heart disease/failure and risk for chronic kidney disease and stroke is direct or a confluence of risk factors is poorly understood.

The increasing prevalence of obesity in the United States and the rest of the world is contributing to our substantial burden of cardiovascular disease including heart disease and congestive heart failure [1–4]. Overnutrition, with our Western diet as a driver of obesity, contributes substantially to a pro-oxidative/inflammatory milieu that promotes alterations in fatty acid, lipid, and glucose metabolism that influence myocardial function and progression of heart failure from diastolic to systolic failure [5]. Progressive heart failure is well documented to be associated with progressive chronic kidney disease (CKD), often referred to as the cardiorenal syndrome (CRS), as well as a prognosticator for cerebrovascular disease (e.g. stroke) [2–4] (fig. 1). Whether the relationship between obesity, heart disease/failure and risk for CKD and stroke is direct or a confluence of risk factors is unknown.

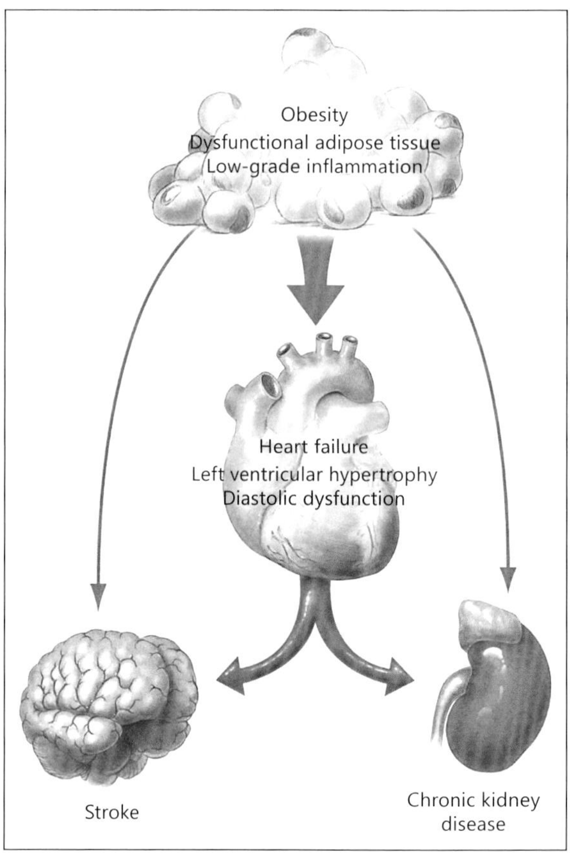

Fig. 1. Obesity is a proinflammatory state that has detrimental effects on multiple organ systems independent of the known risk factors for CVD. The role of obesity in causing cerebrovascular disease and CKD, independently or via pathogenesis of heart failure, is depicted here.

Recent data derived from the National Health and Nutrition Examination Survey (NHANES) support that incident and prevalent obesity in the United States is increasing [1–5]. In the context of cardiovascular disease, obesity has had a disproportionate impact on the adolescent and African-American communities and is thought to contribute annually to approximately 112,000 preventable deaths [6]. In this context there is substantial evidence to support a causal association between obesity and risk for cardiovascular disease (CVD) [7–9]. Data derived from the Framingham and Nurse's Health Study support a continuous, graded relationship between increases in BMI and mortality that began at an approximate BMI >25 as a marker for overweight or obesity [7, 8]. Another report from an Italian cohort suggests a similar relationship between BMI, waist circumference and incident CVD events and all-cause mortality over a 10-year period [9]. Data from this study further suggest that the relationship between BMI and CVD mortality is independent of other metabolic markers such as blood pressure, dysglycemia, serum cholesterol, and triglycerides. Considering that overnutrition conveys this metabolic milieu, a recent meta-analysis further refines this relationship between obesity and CVD and suggests that BMI is an independent risk factor for coronary heart disease [10]. The authors suggest that the confounding elevations in cholesterol and blood pressure introduced in the individual studies may not completely explain the increased risk of heart disease and other comorbidities associated with obesity.

In this regard, obesity predisposes individuals to a large number of comorbidities and increased mortality rates. The risk for coronary heart disease and congestive heart failure (CHF) is clear and recent work highlights an even more complex relationship between obesity, stroke and kidney disease.

Obesity and Risk for CHF

Overnutrition and the development of overweight and obesity is associated with the development of insulin resistance, elevations in blood pressure, dysglycemia, oxidative stress, increased systemic inflammation and alterations in lipids that affect cardiac structure and ultimately function. However, excess body weight in-and-of-itself has been shown to increase both pre- and afterload volume retention, and affect peripheral arterial resistance that enhances pressor-dependent increases in left ventricular (LV) hypertrophy [11]. In turn, the impact that overweight and obesity has on cardiac function has been hard to separate from the elevations in blood pressure, as both eccentric and concentric LV geometric patterns have been described in these conditions that precondition the heart to fail (e.g. CHF) [11, 12].

The evolution of heart failure has been an area of extensive study, but in the context of obesity the pathological factors are incompletely understood. However, the graded risk between increasing obesity and CHF is well recognized and several studies over time have extended our understanding between the association of obesity and heart failure to longitudinal risk [7]. An analysis of 5,881 participants in the Framingham Heart Study, suggests a strong relationship between increases in BMI and an increased risk for heart failure. Following clinical adjustments for diabetes, hypertension, and lipids, for each incremental increase of 1 in BMI, there was 5 and 7% increase in risk for heart failure in men and women, respectively [13]. Preclinical data would suggest the early geometric changes in cardiac structure due to obesity predispose to LV diastolic dysfunction and more recently, data from a Turkish cohort suggest that BMI is an independent predictor of LV diastolic dysfunction [14].

Changes in Myocardium Structure Related to Obesity

Obese individuals tend to have increased LV mass and wall thickness [15]. Our understanding of the effect that obesity has on the myocardial structure and function has evolved overtime. In the early part of 19th century, investigators attributed obesity associated increased weight of heart to epicardial fat deposition. Contrary to this, now it is evident that increased heart weight is largely due to left ventricular hypertrophy. While subject to some controversy, it is generally thought the maladaptive LV structural changes progress with increasing duration and severity of obesity. Initially, the left ventricle undergoes concentric remodeling, which progresses to concentric hypertrophy and ultimately to eccentric hypertrophy if the stress of obesity continues unabated [16]. The progression has been challenged as some have reported a high prevalence of concentric hypertrophy; however, it is unclear if these findings are due to confounding factors like systemic hypertension [15]. Considering that obesity and hypertension coexist and that hypertension is underdiagnosed and often diagnosed late, it will be challenging to design epidemiological studies to answer this question with precision.

Pathogenesis of Metabolic Cardiomyopathy

In states of obesity and chronic over nutrition, the capacity of adipocytes to safely store fat is often exceeded. This leads to hypertrophy and hyperplasia of adipocytes as well as increased fat deposition in the myocardium. Adipocyte hypertrophy is considered a high stress state for the endoplasmic reticulum, and is associated with local hypoxia and pro-inflammatory changes like release of macrophage chemoattractant proteins and infiltration by macrophages [16]. Under stress, the endoplasmic reticulum activates inflammatory pathways that trigger insulin resistance, thereby leading to release of free fatty acids in plasma. An increase in circulating free fatty acids is associated with ectopic deposition of fat in the myocardium through downregulation of peroxisome proliferator-activated receptor-α in rodent models [17]. It is unclear if these findings can be extrapolated verbatim to human cardiomyocytes as well, but it does appear that there is a mismatch between the fatty acid supply and utilization in states of insulin resistance, which promotes steatosis in the myocardium. The problem is further accentuated by the decrease in maximal fatty acid oxidation capacity of the mitochondria in heart muscle, in the presence of an increased supply of fats [18].

Even though a healthy human heart predominantly uses fatty acids for ATP production during the normal physiological state, it can rapidly switch to glucose during times of stress [19]. The ability of the heart to switch between different substrates depending on the physiological and pathological stressors, substrate availability and oxygen supply is crucial for its optimal performance [19]. Decreased insulin sensitivity is associated with the decreased ability of the heart to switch to glucose use at times of stress, e.g. during ischemia, heart failure or pathological hypertrophy [20]. In this regard, Peterson et al. [21] demonstrated that obese females had higher myocardial oxygen consumption, and increasing BMI was a predictor of decreasing efficiency of myocardium in oxygen utilization. Decreased efficiency of heart in states of stress is a hallmark of early heart failure.

Recent work supports that mitochondria in the myocardium of people with diabetes might be a source of increased reactive oxygen species (ROS) [18]. These ROS can oxidize and damage intracellular lipids and proteins. ROS are also known to damage mitochondrial DNA and further impair mitochondrial respiration [19]. The changes in myocardial substrate utilization, ultrastructure, calcium handling, mitochondrial uncoupling, increased ROS production, lipotoxicity, local inflammation, and apoptosis have been implicated in pathogenesis of diabetic or metabolic cardiomyopathy. The understanding of this entity is far from complete. More studies are required to unravel the complicated mechanistic details.

Obesity, Heart Failure and Stroke

Heart failure has been long established as risk predictor for future CVD events. In this context, previous work suggests that the risk of stroke among heart failure patients is almost seven times higher than in the general population [22, 23]. The link between obesity and heart failure is emerging; however, an often neglected consideration in the obesity epidemic is the preponderance of stroke. It is estimated that approximately 1 of every 15 deaths or approximately 700,000 people experience a new or recurrent stroke each year [23]. In this context, stroke is the third leading cause of death after heart disease and current thought lends to the perception that the increase in stroke events is driven by increasing incident and prevalent hypertension, diabetes, or atrial fibrillation [23–26]. However, when considering known predictors of stroke including diabetes mellitus, hypertension, dyslipidemia and tobacco use, the importance of obesity in driving the recent increases in incident stroke becomes evident.

Data from several recent meta-analyses would support this trend in obesity and risk for stroke [27, 28]. One recent meta-analysis including two million participants suggests that there is a graded positive relationship between obesity and incident ischemic stroke [27]. Another meta-analysis from a Japanese population demonstrates a very specific linear association between increases in BMI and ischemic and hemorrhagic stroke [28]. Interestingly, this study highlights a positive association between progressive increases in BMI within the normal and overweight range (20–29) and risk of CVD. An analysis of the Framingham study also pointed to the positive association between overweight (BMI 25–29.9) and relative risk of hypertension and cardiovascular sequelae [29]. Further analyses of Framingham data indicate that abdominal obesity after clinical adjustments for diabetes, hypertension and other CVD risk confounders, independently increases the risk for stroke, heart failure and all-cause mortality in men [30]. This would highlight obesity as a central driver of the heart failure-stroke risk.

Most concerning in understanding this relationship between obesity, heart failure and stroke are the increasing adolescence obesity rates. Data from this meta-analysis of 63 studies supports that obese children are at increased risk for type 2 diabetes, hypertension, dyslipidemia and future risk for heart failure and stroke [31]. These data would further suggest that if these children lost weight, future CVD risk would be attenuated. Cumulative data on obesity and cardiovascular risk would suggest weight loss in general would improve risk parameters such as diabetes, high blood pressure, and lipids, but long term work has yet to elucidate the beneficial impact of weight loss on hard cardiovascular endpoints

Obesity-Related Heart Failure as the Intermediate in the Cerebrorenal Connection

Congruent with an obesity epidemic, there is an exponential increase in chronic kidney disease (CKD) in the general population. Similar to the risk observed with increases in BMI and cardiovascular outcomes such as heart failure and stroke, there exists a graded relationship between increases in BMI and incident CKD and microalbuminuria [32, 33]. This is illustrated over numerous population-based studies estimating the relative risk for CKD in relation to increases in BMI ≥25. This association holds true even after clinical adjustments for diabetes and hypertension [32, 33]. In this regard, BMI ≥30 in males and BMI ≥35 in females is associated with a 3- to 4-fold increased risk for CKD. The risk between obesity and CKD is augmented in the presence of other CKD risk factors such as diabetes and hypertension.

It is well accepted that there exists a graded relationship between reductions in estimated glomerular filtration rate or increases in proteinuria and CVD morbidity and mortality including heart failure and stroke [34, 35]. However, it is increasingly recognized this relationship is bidirectional in nature and is often referred to as the CRS [5]. When considering metabolic risk factors for both heart and kidney disease such as diabetes, hypertension, dyslipidemia or aging, we refer to this as the CRS. The physiology of the CRS involves a complex intersection of reductions in renal perfusion pressure, alterations in tubuloglomerular feedback and altered intrarenal hemodynamics from progressive heart failure. In turn, neurohormonal systems such as inappropriate activation of the sympathetic nervous system and renin-angiotensin-aldosterone system that arise from both heart failure and kidney disease integrate the impact that obesity has on CVD including stroke.

While we know much about the relationship between obesity, heart failure and kidney disease, there is increasing interest in how this relates to cerebrovascular disease. Recent work would suggest that the risk for stroke including transient ischemic attacks is inordinately high in the presence of CKD compared to other cardiovascular outcomes [36, 37]. However, findings from these studies appear to hold true only for those with CKD due to diabetes or hypertension. Data from The Atherosclerosis Risk in Communities (ARIC) study would suggest the risk for stroke is further modified by the presence of anemia [37] whereas data from a Japanese cohort suggests this relationship exists independent of other effect modifiers like diabetes, hypertension or anemia [38]. In essence, these collective findings suggest that perhaps CKD accelerates atherosclerosis in the presence of other cardiovascular risk factors, yet it is unclear whether the presence CKD alone may be insufficient as an independent risk factor for stroke.

Conclusions

In summary, there is an emerging interest in the effect that obesity has on heart failure as a mediator of cardiovascular outcomes including stroke and kidney disease. Overnutrition with our Western diet contributes substantially to a pro oxidative/inflammatory milieu that promotes alterations in fatty acid, lipid and glucose metabolism that influence myocardial function and the progression of heart failure from diastolic to systolic failure. In this regard, progressive heart failure is well documented to be associated with CKD referred to as the CRS, and is a significant prognosticator for cerebrovascular disease (e.g. stroke). Whether this relationship between obesity, heart disease/failure and risk for CKD and stroke is direct or a confluence of risk factors is unknown.

References

1 Flegal KM, Carroll MD, Kit BK, Ogden CL: Prevalence of obesity and trends in the distribution of body mass index among US adults, 1999–2010. JAMA 2012;307:491–497.

2 Appelros P, Nydevik I, Seiger Å, Terént A: Predictors of severe stroke: influence of preexisting dementia and cardiac disorders. Stroke 2002;33:2357–2362.

3 Ejerblad E, Fored CM, Lindblad P, Fryzek J, McLaughlin JK, Nyrén O: Obesity and risk for chronic renal failure. J Am Soc Nephrol 2006;17:1695–1702.

4 Hsu CY, McCulloch CE, Iribarren C, Darbinian J, Go AS: Body mass index and risk for end-stage renal disease. Ann Intern Med 2006;144:21–28.

5 Sowers JR, Whaley-Connell A, Hayden MR: The role of overweight and obesity in the cardiorenal syndrome. Cardiorenal Med 2011;1: 5–12.

6 US Department of Health and Human Services: The Surgeon General's Vision for a Healthy and Fit Nation. Rockville, US Department of Health and Human Services, Office of the Surgeon General, 2010.

7 Manson JE, Willett WC, Stampfer MJ, Colditz GA, Hunter DJ, Hankinson SE, Hennekens CH, Speizer FE: Body weight and mortality among women. N Engl J Med 1995;333:677–685.

8 Wilson PW, D'Agostino RB, Sullivan L, Parise H, Kannel WB: Overweight and obesity as determinants of cardiovascular risk: the Framingham experience. Arch Intern Med 2002;162:1867–1872.

9 Bombelli M, Facchetti R, Fodri D, Brambilla G, Sega R, Grassi G, Mancia G: Impact of body mass index and waist circumference on the cardiovascular risk and all-cause death in a general population: data from the PAMELA study. Nutr Metab Cardiovasc Dis 2012, Epub ahead of print.

10 Bogers RP, Bemelmans WJ, Hoogenveen RT, Boshuizen HC, Woodward M, Knekt P, van Dam RM, Hu FB, Visscher TL, Menotti A, Thorpe RJ Jr, Jamrozik K, Calling S, Strand BH, Shipley MJ, for the BMI-CHD Collaboration Investigators: Association of overweight with increased risk of coronary heart disease partly independent of blood pressure and cholesterol levels: a meta-analysis of 21 cohort studies including more than 300,000 persons. Arch Intern Med 2007;167:1720–1728.

11 Alpert MA: Obesity cardiomyopathy: pathophysiology and evolution of the clinical syndrome. Am J Med Sci 2001;321:225–236.

12 Turkbey EB, McClelland RL, Kronmal RA, Burke GL, Bild DE, Tracy RP, Arai AE, Lima JA, Bluemke DA: The impact of obesity on the left ventricle: the Multi-Ethnic Study of Atherosclerosis (MESA). JACC Cardiovasc Imaging 2010;3:266–274.

13 Kenchaiah S, Evans JC, Levy D, Wilson PW, Benjamin EJ, Larson MG, Kannel WB, Vasan RS: Obesity and the risk of heart failure. N Engl J Med 2002;347:305–313.

14 Cil H, Bulur S, Turker Y, Kaya A, Alemdar R, Karabacak A, Aslantas Y, Ekinozu I, Albayrak S, Ozhan H, MELEN Investigators: Impact of body mass index on left ventricular diastolic dysfunction. Echocardiography 2012;29:647–651.

15 Alpert MA, Chan EJ: Left ventricular morphology and diastolic function in severe obesity: current views. Rev Esp Cardiol (Engl) 2012;65:1–3.

16 Lionetti L, Mollica MP, Lombardi A, Cavaliere G, Gifuni G, Barletta A: From chronic overnutrition to insulin resistance: the role of fat-storing capacity and inflammation. Nutr Metab Cardiovasc Dis 2009;19:146–152.

17 van de Weijer T, Schrauwen-Hinderling VB, Schrauwen P: Lipotoxicity in type 2 diabetic cardiomyopathy. Cardiovasc Res 2011;92: 10–18.

18 Anderson EJ, Kypson AP, Rodriguez E, Anderson CA, Lehr EJ, Neufer PD: Substrate-specific derangements in mitochondrial metabolism and redox balance in the atrium of the type 2 diabetic human heart. J Am Coll Cardiol 2009;54:1891–1898.

19 Duncan JG: Mitochondrial dysfunction in diabetic cardiomyopathy. Biochim Biophys Acta 2011;1813:1351–1359.

20 Zhou YT, Grayburn P, Karim A, Shimabukuro M, Higa M, Baetens D, Orci L, Unger RH: Lipotoxic heart disease in obese rats: implications for human obesity. Proc Natl Acad Sci USA 2000;97:1784–1789.

21 Peterson LR, Herrero P, Schechtman KB, Racette SB, Waggoner AD, Kisrieva-Ware Z, Dence C, Klein S, Marsala J, Meyer T, Gropler RJ: Effect of obesity and insulin resistance on myocardial substrate metabolism and efficiency in young women. Circulation 2004;109: 2191–2196.

22 Witt BJ, Gami AS, Ballman KV, Brown RD Jr, Meverden RA, Jacobsen SJ, Roger VL: The incidence of ischemic stroke in chronic heart failure: a meta-analysis. J Card Fail 2007;13: 489–496.
23 Thom T, Haase N, Rosamond W, Howard VJ, Rumsfeld J, Manolio T, Zheng ZJ, Flegal K, O'Donnell C, Kittner S, Lloyd-Jones D, Goff DC Jr, Hong Y, Adams R, Friday G, Furie K, Gorelick P, Kissela B, Marler J, Meigs J, Roger V, Sidney S, Sorlie P, Steinberger J, Wasserthiel-Smoller S, Wilson M, Wolf P: Heart disease and stroke statistics: 2006 update – a report from the American Heart Association Statistics Committee and Stroke Statistics Subcommittee. Circulation 2006;113:e85–e151.
24 Wolf PA, D'Agostino RB, Kannel WB, Bonita R, Belanger AJ: Cigarette smoking as a risk factor for stroke: the Framingham study. JAMA 1988;259:1025–1029.
25 Wolf PA, Abbott RD, Kannel WB: Atrial fibrillation as an independent risk factor for stroke: the Framingham study. Stroke 1991; 22:983–988.
26 Seshadri S, Beiser A, Kelly-Hayes M, Kase CS, Au R, Kannel WB, Wolf PA: The lifetime risk of stroke: estimates from the Framingham Study. Stroke 2006;37:345–350.
27 Strazzullo P, D'Elia L, Cairella G, Garbagnati F, Cappuccio FP, Scalfi L: Excess body weight and incidence of stroke: meta-analysis of prospective studies with 2 million participants. Stroke 2010;41:e418–e426.
28 Yatsuya H, Toyoshima H, Yamagishi K, Tamakoshi K, Taguri M, Harada A, Ohashi Y, Kita Y, Naito Y, Yamada M, Tanabe N, Iso H, Ueshima H, Japan Arteriosclerosis Longitudinal Study (JALS) Group: Body mass index and risk of stroke and myocardial infarction in a relatively lean population: meta-analysis of 16 Japanese cohorts using individual data. Circ Cardiovasc Qual Outcomes 2010;3:498–505.
29 Wilson PW, D'Agostino RB, Sullivan L, Parise H, Kannel WB: Overweight and obesity as determinants of cardiovascular risk: the Framingham experience. Arch Intern Med 2002;162:1867–1872.
30 Kannel WB, Cupples LA, Ramaswami R, Stokes J, Kreger BE, Higgins M: Regional obesity and risk of cardiovascular disease: the Framingham Study. J Clin Epidemiol 1991; 44:183–190.
31 Friedemann C, Heneghan C, Mahtani K, Thompson M, Perera R, Ward AM: Cardiovascular disease risk in healthy children and its association with body mass index: systematic review and meta-analysis. BMJ 2012; 345:e4759.
32 Ejerblad E, Fored CM, Lindblad P, Fryzek J, McLaughlin JK, Nyrén O: Obesity and risk for chronic renal failure. J Am Soc Nephrol 2006;17:1695–1702.
33 Yamagata K, Ishida K, Sairenchi T, Takahashi H, Ohba S, Shiigai T, Narita M, Koyama A: Risk factors for chronic kidney disease in a community-based population: a 10-year follow-up study. Kidney Int 2007; 71:159–166.
34 Sowers JR, Whaley-Connell A, Hayden MR: The role of overweight and obesity in the cardiorenal syndrome. Cardiorenal Med 2011;1: 5–12.
35 Dhingra R, Gaziano JM, Djoussé L: Chronic kidney disease and the risk of heart failure in men. Circ Heart Fail 2011;4:138–144.
36 Koren-Morag N, Goldbourt U, Tanne D: Renal dysfunction and risk of ischemic stroke or TIA in patients with cardiovascular disease. Neurology 2006;67:224–228.
37 Abramson JL, Jurkovitz CT, Vaccarino V, Weintraub WS, McClellan W: Chronic kidney disease, anemia, and incident stroke in a middle-aged, community-based population: the ARIC study. Kidney Int 2003;64:610–615.
38 Nakayama M, Metoki H, Terawaki H, Ohkubo T, Kikuya M, Sato T, Nakayama K, Asayama K, Inoue R, Hashimoto J, Totsune K, Hoshi H, Ito S, Imai Y: Kidney dysfunction as a risk factor for first symptomatic stroke events in a general Japanese population: the Ohasama study. Nephrol Dial Transplant 2007;22:1910–1915.

James R. Sowers, MD
Diabetes and Cardiovascular Center of Excellence
Columbia School of Medicine, University of Missouri
One Hospital Drive, Columbia, MO 65212 (USA)
E-Mail sowersj@health.missouri.edu

Risk of Clinical and Subclinical Brain Damage in Kidney Disease

Toyoda K (ed): Brain, Stroke and Kidney.
Contrib Nephrol. Basel, Karger, 2013, vol 179, pp 24–34 (DOI: 10.1159/000346719)

Subclinical Cerebral Abnormalities in Chronic Kidney Disease

Hiroshi Yao[a] · Yuki Takashima[a] · Manabu Hashimoto[a] · Akira Uchino[b] · Takefumi Yuzuriha[a]

[a]Center for Emotional and Behavioral Disorders, National Hospital Organization Hizen Psychiatric Center, Saga, and [b]Department of Radiology, Saitama Medical University International Medical Center, Saitama, Japan

Abstract

Background and Purpose: Impaired kidney function or chronic kidney disease (CKD), as measured by estimated glomerular filtration rate (eGFR), is associated with incident stroke risk. However, few studies have examined the relationship between CKD and subclinical cerebral abnormalities. ***Methods:*** We examined 675 elderly subjects (mean age 69.9 years), who were living independently at home without apparent dementia, using magnetic resonance imaging. Serum creatinine values, measured by the enzymatic method, were used for the Japanese equation of eGFR. ***Results:*** Subclinical lacunar infarction, deep white matter lesions, and periventricular hyperintensities were detected in 88 (13.0%), 240 (35.6%) and 158 (23.4%) of the 675 participants, respectively. In the forward stepwise method of logistic analysis, age (OR 2.081/10, 95% CI 1.541–2.810), hypertension (OR 3.656, 95% CI 2.184–6.119), diabetes mellitus (OR 1.961, 95% CI 1.007–3.820), alcohol intake (OR 2.130, 95% CI 1.283–3.535), and eGFR <45 ml/min/1.73 m^2 were significant factors concerning subclinical lacunar infarction. CKD defined as eGFR <60 ml/min/1.73 m^2 was not significantly associated with subclinical lacunar infarction. Decreased eGFR was not a significant factor associated with white matter lesions (WMLs). Age (OR 2.781/10, 95% CI 2.252–3.435), hypertension (OR 1.746, 95% CI 1.231–2.477), diabetes mellitus (OR 1.854, 95% CI 1.070–3.213), but not eGFR were significant factors concerning WMLs. ***Conclusions:*** The present study showed that community dwelling elderly subjects with late stage 3 CKD were at high risk for prevalent subclinical lacunar infarction. The identification of CKD-specific modifiable risk factors for SBI and WMLs is of increased importance for prevention of subclinical brain ischemic lesions.

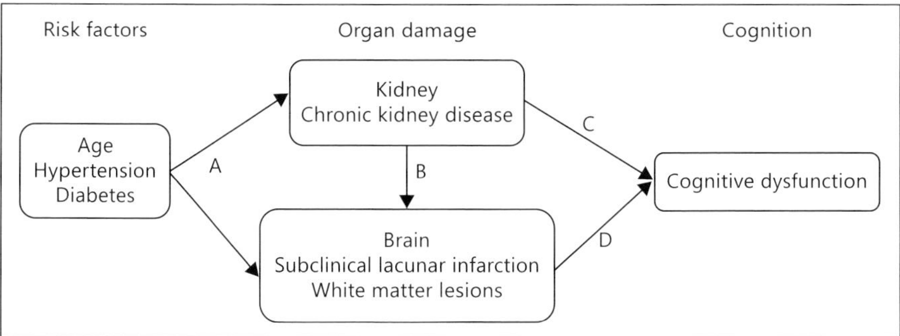

Fig. 1. CKD and silent or subclinical brain ischemic lesions share many common risk factors (A), most studies demonstrated that CKD increases the risk of SBI and WMLs independent of classical vascular risk factors (B). Our previous study revealed frontal lobe dysfunction associated with CKD and independent of subclinical lacunar infarction (C). Subclinical brain ischemic lesions such as silent brain infarction and white matter lesions are the basis for cognitive dysfunction (D). Future studies should elucidate CKD-specific mechanisms (B and C) to prevent subclinical brain ischemic lesions and cognitive dysfunction.

Chronic kidney disease (CKD) is becoming a common disease. The prevalence of CKD in elderly persons aged 64 years or older varied from 23.4 to 35.8% [1]. In a large community-based sample of participants free of kidney disease at baseline, multivariable predictors of the development of kidney disease included diabetes, hypertension, obesity, smoking, low HDL-cholesterol level, and a mild reduction in estimated glomerular filtration rate (eGFR) [2]. Among a random sample of 25,821 subjects, 94 cases with end-stage renal disease were identified during a mean follow-up of 26.5 years: male gender, hypertension, diabetes, and obesity were independent risk factors for end-stage renal disease, and diabetes was the most powerful predictor [3]. Subjects with CKD are clearly at risk for development of cardiovascular diseases [4, 5]. The Chronic Kidney Disease Prognosis Consortium reported the results of a collaborative meta-analysis, including 1.23 million participants, with a median follow-up of 7.9 years and showed that eGFR and albuminuria were associated with all-cause mortality and cardiovascular mortality independent of each other and traditional cardiovascular risk factors [4]. Microalbuminuria and low GFR were strongly associated with incident stroke risk [6, 7].

Recent studies have proposed that CKD is an independent risk factor for cognitive impairment, dementia and vascular cognitive impairment (fig. 1). A systematic review revealed that most, not all, cross-sectional and longitudinal studies suggested an association between cognitive impairment and CKD [8]. However, the mechanisms of cognitive impairment in subjects with CKD are unclear. Most studies support the association between CKD and subclinical ischemic brain lesions such as silent brain infarction (SBI) and white matter lesions (WMLs) [9]. To our knowledge, no study has reported an association between cerebral microbleeds, another type or cerebral small vessel disease, and CKD in the general population. Although vascular factors and/or cerebral ischemic lesions may be the basis for cognitive decline (i.e. vascular cognitive impairment) in subjects with CKD, our previous study failed to reveal an independent association of CKD with subclinical ischemic brain lesions [10]. Our previous study was restricted to subjects aged 60 years or older, and those who received cognitive function tests. Therefore, we extended the analysis by inclusion of subjects without cognitive function tests to examine the relationship among subclinical MRI lesions, vascular risk factors, and CKD.

Subjects and Methods

Participants

Between 1997 and 2011, we randomly contacted approximately 1,200 inhabitants, aged 40 years or older, living in the rural community of Sefuri village, Saga, Japan, through the village office information service. For this study, 712 participants aged 50–89 years with brain MRI and kidney function measurements were initially included. These subjects were living independently at home without apparent dementia. A total of 37 cases were excluded because of claustrophobia or contraindications for MRI (n = 8), a history of stroke (n = 15), brain tumor (n = 3), psychiatric disorders including depression (n = 4), a history of head trauma (n = 2), and insufficient clinical information (n = 5). Subjects with a history of minor stroke and normal neurological examination upon MRI imaging were included. Consequently, we enrolled 675 subjects in the present study.

The National Hospital Organization Hizen Psychiatric Center Institutional Review Board approved the study (No. 15-1), and written informed consent was obtained from all subjects.

Definition of Vascular Risk Factors

Fasting blood samples were taken in the morning, and general hematology and biochemistry tests were performed. Blood pressure was measured in the sitting position by the standard cuff method after a 5-min rest. Vascular risk factors were defined as previously described [10]. Briefly, arterial hypertension was considered present if a subject had a history of repeated blood pressure recordings above 140/90 mm Hg or the subject was being treated for hypertension. Diabetes mellitus was defined as fasting plasma glucose greater than 7.77 mmol/l and/or HbA1c greater than 6.0% or a previous diagnosis of diabetes mellitus. Hyperlipidemia was defined by either total serum cholesterol concentration greater than 5.69 mmol/l or current treatment for hyperlipidemia. Left ventricular hypertrophy, ST depression, and atrial fibrillation were measured on 12 lead electrocardiograms. In the present study, we defined alcohol intake as one drink or more per week, and former drinkers were considered nondrinkers in the present study. Smoking was defined as present if the subject smoked at least an average of 10 cigarettes per day.

Serum creatinine values, measured by the enzymatic method, were used for the new Japanese equation of eGFR modified from the Modification of Diet in Renal Disease (MDRD) Study equation: eGFR (ml/min/1.73 m^2) = 194 × (serum creatinine [mg/dl])$^{-1.094}$ × (age)$^{-0.287}$ × (0.739 if female) [11]. GFR levels were classified as ≥90, 60–89, 45–59 and <45 ml/min/1.73 m^2 according to the standard guidelines and to Chou et al. [12].

Assessment of MRI Findings

The combination of T1-weighted (T1WI), T2-weighted (T2WI), and fluid attenuated inversion recovery (FLAIR) images is required to accurately detect both SBI and WMLs [13]. Therefore, T1WI, T2WI, and FLAIR images were obtained with a slice thickness of 6 mm with a 1-mm interslice gap as previously described [10]. SBI appeared as low signal intensities on T1-weighted images, and their size was 5 mm or larger. We differentiated enlarged perivascular spaces from SBI based on their location, shape and size. The WMLs were defined as isointense to normal brain parenchyma on T1-weighted images, but were high signal intensity areas on T2-weighted images. These were classified into either deep white matter lesions (DWMLs) or periventricular hyperintensities (PVHs). For statistical analyses, we used combined DWML and PVH grades to evaluate WMLs. All scans were reviewed independently by 2 authors (H.Y. and A.U.) who were blinded to all clinical data. In the case of disagreement between the raters, a consensus reading was held.

Statistical Analysis

Summary statistics of clinical variables were given as the mean ± SD. For the univariate analysis, the Mann-Whitney U test for continuous variables, and the χ^2 test for categorical variables were used. We chose the variables for entry into the multivariate analysis based on the clinical and neuroradiological findings after univariate testing. Multivariate analysis was done using the forward stepwise method of logistic analysis. A significance level of 0.05 was used in all analyses. The data were analyzed with the IBM SPSS Statistics 18 software for Windows (SPSS Japan Inc.).

Results

The subjects were 271 men and 404 women with a mean age of 69.9 (range 50–89) years (table 1). Hypertension was present in 271 subjects (40.1%). The prevalence of diabetes mellitus, hyperlipidemia, and ischemic heart disease was 10.7, 24.4 and 6.8%, respectively. The mean value of serum creatinine was 61.9 μmol/l (range 35.4–450.8 μmol/l), and the frequency of GFR <60 ml/min/1.73 m^2 was 15.9%. Subclinical lacunar infarction, DWMLs and PVHs were detected in 88 (13.0%), 240 (35.6%) and 158 (23.4%) of the 675 participants, respectively. Both DWMLs and PVHs were gradually increased with advanced stages of CKD (fig. 2). In contrast, the prevalence of subclinical lacunar infarction was increased steeply in the late stage 3 CKD group (42.9%) compared with early stages of CKD (7.4 to 15.1%).

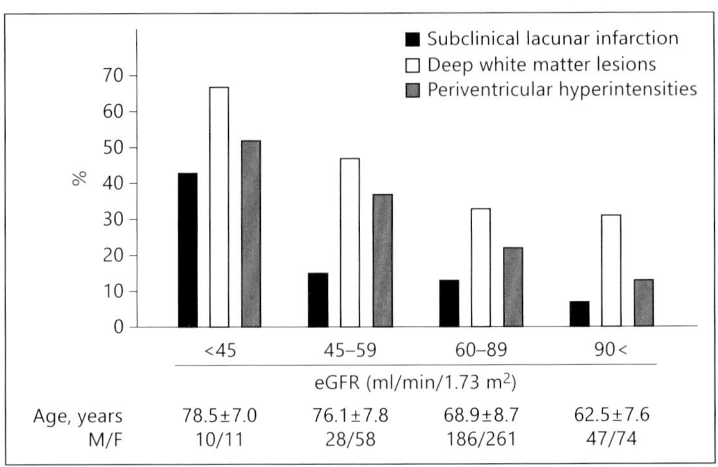

Fig. 2. The prevalence of subclinical lacunar infarction, deep white matter lesions and periventricular hyperintensities in different stages of CKD. Both deep white matter lesions and periventricular hyperintensities were gradually increased with advanced stages of CKD. The prevalence of subclinical lacunar infarction was strikingly elevated in subjects with late stage 3 CKD group compared with early stages of CKD.

Table 1. Characteristics of the study population

	Total cohort (n = 675)
Age, years	69.9±9.3
Women	404 (59.9)
BMI, kg/m^2	23.0±3.4
Hypertension	271 (40.1)
Systolic BP, mm Hg	140.3±22.5
Diastolic BP, mm Hg	80.9±10.7
Diabetes mellitus	72 (10.7)
Hyperlipidemia	165 (24.4)
Alcohol	244 (36.1)
Smoking	230 (34.1)
Ischemic heart disease	46 (6.8)
Atrial fibrillation	16 (2.4)
Hematocrit, fraction of 1.00	0.40±0.05
Albumin, g/l	43±3
Fasting blood glucose, mmol/l	5.52±1.43
Total cholesterol, mmol/l	5.15±0.93
HDL cholesterol, mmol/l	1.59±0.42
Uric acid, μmol/l	297±83
Creatinine, μmol/l	61.9±26.5
eGFR, ml/min/1.73 m^2	74.5±16.2

Data are presented as n (%) or mean ± SD.

Table 2. Possible risk factors for subclinical lacunar infarction

	Model 1			Model 2		
	OR	95% CI	p	OR	95% CI	p
Age (/10 years)	2.081	1.541–2.810	0.000	2.192	1.631–2.945	0.000
Sex	–	–	–	–	–	–
Hypertension	3.656	2.184–6.119	0.000	3.729	2.233–6.228	0.000
Diabetes mellitus	1.961	1.007–3.820	0.0048	2.040	1.053–3.951	0.035
Alcohol	2.130	1.283–3.535	0.003	2.098	1.269–3.467	0.004
Smoking	–	–	–	–	–	–
eGFR <45 ml/min/1.73 m^2	2.645	0.981–7.128	0.054			
eGFR <60 ml/min/1.73 m^2				–	–	–

In the forward stepwise method of logistic analysis, age (OR 2.081/10 years, 95% CI 1.541–2.810), hypertension (OR 3.656, 95% CI 2.184–6.119), diabetes mellitus (OR 1.961, 95% CI 1.007–3.820), alcohol intake (OR 2.130, 95% CI 1.283–3.535), and eGFR <45 ml/min/1.73 m^2 were significant factors concerning subclinical lacunar infarction (table 2, model 1). CKD defined as eGFR <60 ml/min/1.73 m^2 was not significantly associated with subclinical lacunar infarction (table 2, model 2).

With regard to WMLs, age (OR 2.781/10 years, 95% CI 2.252–3.435), hypertension (OR 1.746, 95% CI 1.231–2.477), diabetes mellitus (OR 1.854, 95% CI 1.070–3.213) were significant factors concerning WMLs. Decreased eGFR was not a significant factor associated with WMLs.

Discussion

The present study showed that classical risk factors (i.e. age, hypertension and diabetes mellitus) were independently associated with both subclinical lacunar infarction, and WMLs. These classic vascular risk factors are also the predictors for CKD [2, 3]. However, only advanced stage of CKD was associated with subclinical lacunar infarction but not with WMLs in the present study. A close relationship has been established between small vessel disease in brain and kidney [14]. The brain and kidney are unique in that these organs are perfused throughout systolic and diastolic by pulsatile flow. In particular, strain vessels such as juxtamedullary afferent arterioles in the kidney and small perforating arteries in the brain are exposed to an unusually high pressure [15]. Therefore, both – brain and kidney – may be victims of common vascular risk factors. However, it is not clear whether CKD further aggravates subclinical brain lesions beyond the classical risk factors.

Table 3. Association of CKD and subclinical brain lesions on MRI

Author	Year	Subjects	Mean age, years	Number of participants	Kidney function	Association of CKD with		Vascular risk factors further adjusted in addition to age and sex
						SBI	WMLs	
Seliger et al. [19]: Cardiovascular Health Study	2005	general population	75.0	2,784	cystatin C	+	NA	SBP, DBP, DM, smoking, and medication
Khatri et al. [17]: North Manhattan Study	2007	general population	70	615	Ccr, eGFR	NA	+	HT, DM, IHD, and homocysteine
Ikram et al. [18]: Rotterdam Study	2008	general population	73.4	484	Ccr	NS	+	SBP, DBP, DM, smoking, CRP, homocysteine, TC, HDL, IHD, and medication
Wada et al. [20]	2008	general population	61, 70–72*	625	eGFR	+	+	HT, DM, TC/HDL ratio, and smoking
Kobayashi et al. [22]	2009	CKD, HT	63.5	375	eGFR	+	+	SBP, IHD, smoking, hemoglobin, and TC
Otani et al. [21]: Ohasama Study	2010	general population	66.4	1,008	Ccr	+	NS	24-h SBP, DM, hyperlipidemia, smoking, drinking, IHD, and medication
Shima et al. [23]	2011	CKD	60.7	324	eGFR	+	+	SBP, DBP, PP, DM, LDL, hemoglobin, and medication
Chou et al. [12]	2011	general population	52.5	1,312	eGFR	+	NA	HT, DM, and carotid plaque

Ccr = Creatinine clearance with the Cockcroft-Gault equation; SBI = silent brain infarction; WMLs = white matter lesions; HT = hypertension; PP = pulse pressure; DM = diabetes mellitus; IHD = ischemic heart disease; TC = total cholesterol; HDL = HDL cholesterol; LDL = LDL cholesterol; CRP = C-reactive protein; NA = not available; NS = not significant.
* Subjects at specific ages were invited.

One major limitation of this study relates to its cross-sectional study design, which limits the interpretation of our results with respect to cause and effect, particularly CKD as a presumed prerequisite for subsequent cerebral ischemic lesions. Also, neither urinary albumin nor cystatin C was measured in the present study, which may have limited the evaluation of kidney function. It is, however, noteworthy that estimates of GFR are the best overall indices of kidney function [16]. The advantages of the current study are the inclusion of a relatively large number of community-dwelling subjects and the use of MRI. In particular, structural brain imaging with MRI is indispensable for assessing the relationship between subclinical cerebral abnormalities and CKD.

Although there is mounting evidence that CKD increases the risk of cerebrovascular disease or stroke [4–7], few studies have examined the relationship between CKD and subclinical cerebral abnormalities (table 3) [12, 17–23]. The

Northern Manhattan Study and the Rotterdam Scan Study found that subjects with CKD, defined by reduced creatinine clearance or eGFR, had a greater burden of white matter hyperintensity volumes after adjusting for confounders, such as vascular risk factors [17, 18]. Likewise, in community-dwelling elderly subjects, the association between the presence of CKD and lacunar infarction or moderate WMLs was statistically significant even after adjustment for conventional cardiovascular risk factors, suggesting that CKD was an independent risk factor for cerebral small vessel disease [12, 19, 20]. Most of these studies used eGFR or creatinine clearance for the evaluation of kidney function. However, the Cardiovascular Health Study showed that increasing prevalence of SBI was associated independently with increasing quintiles of cystatin C range, whereas the associations between serum creatinine or eGFR and SBI were U-shaped [19]. CKD was independently associated with SBI and WMLs in elderly subjects with CKD or essential hypertension [22 and Nephrol Dial Transplant 2009;24: 2005–2007 (author reply)]. In predialysis CKD patients, decreased kidney function was an independent factor associated with SBI and PVHs [23]. Taken together, CKD appears to independently increase the risk of SBI and/or WMLs in most of the studies in table 3.

In the present study, however, the association between late stage 3 CKD and subclinical lacunar infarction was marginally significant. Among subjects with stages 1–3, the SBI risk increased only in late stage 3 CKD even after adjusting for age, gender, hypertension, diabetes, and carotid plaque [12]. Kobayashi et al. [22] also demonstrated a significant association between SBI and the group of eGFR <30 ml/min/1.73 m^2. These studies including ours may indicate that detrimental effects of CKD on subclinical ischemic brain lesions are especially evident at more advanced stages of CKD. In other words, CKD-specific mechanisms responsible for the development of SBI and WMLs may exert detrimental effects beyond the classical vascular risk factors only in advanced CKD.

There are several biologically plausible mechanisms through which CKD could result in subclinical MRI lesions. Novel and nontraditional risk factors, such as inflammation, oxidative stress, endothelial dysfunction, and altered levels of adipokines, involved in the vascular damage in CKD have been described [24]. Inflammatory and procoagulant pathways and asymmetric dimethylarginine, an endogenous inhibitor of nitric oxide synthase, might be important mediators leading to the increased cardiovascular risks of patients with CKD [25, 26]. High rather than low adiponectin, an adipocyte-derived protein with anti-inflammatory, anti-atherogenic and insulin sensitizing activity were predictors of all-cause and cerebrovascular mortality in patients with stage 3 to 4 CKD [27]. There have been no interventional studies with adiponectin on cardiovascular outcome; thus, it remains unclear whether adiponectin confers vascular protection [28]. Although folic acid supplementation significantly improved cognitive function [29], the renal Heart Outcomes Prevention Evaluation (HOPE)-2 study recently reported that active treatment with B vitamins lowered homocysteine in participants with CKD but had no effect on cardiovascular outcomes [30].

In conclusion, the present study showed that late stage 3 CKD was independently associated with subclinical lacunar infarction in community-dwelling healthy subjects. Although CKD and silent or subclinical brain ischemic lesions share many common risk factors, most studies demonstrated that CKD increases the risk of SBI and WMLs independent of classical vascular risk factors. Therefore, the identification of CKD-specific modifiable risk factors for SBI and WMLs is of increased importance for prevention of subclinical brain ischemic lesions.

Acknowledgements

We wish to express special thanks to T. Ninomiya, MD, for his valuable advice during the course of this study. We also thank T. Muto, and K. Akashi for technical assistance with the laboratory examinations and MRI scanning and K. Muto for registration of participants.

References

1 Zhang QL, Rothenbacher D: Prevalence of chronic kidney disease in population-based studies: systematic review. BMC Publ Health 2008;8:117.
2 Fox CS, Larson MG, Leip EP, Culleton B, Wilson PW, Levy D: Predictors of new-onset kidney disease in a community-based population. JAMA 2004;291:844–850.
3 Kastarinen M, Juutilainen A, Kastarinen H, Salomaa V, Karhapää P, Tuomilehto J, Grönhagen-Riska C, Jousilahti P, Finne P: Risk factors for end-stage renal disease in a community-based population: 26-year follow-up of 25,821 men and women in eastern Finland. J Intern Med 2010;267:612–620.
4 Chronic Kidney Disease Prognosis Consortium, Matsushita K, van der Velde M, Astor BC, Woodward M, Levey AS, de Jong PE, Coresh J, Gansevoort RT: Association of estimated glomerular filtration rate and albuminuria with all-cause and cardiovascular mortality in general population cohorts: a collaborative meta-analysis. Lancet 2010;375:2073–2081.
5 Ninomiya T, Kiyohara Y, Tokuda Y, Doi Y, Arima H, Harada A, Ohashi Y, Ueshima H; Japan Arteriosclerosis Longitudinal Study Group: Impact of kidney disease and blood pressure on the development of cardiovascular disease: an overview from the Japan Arteriosclerosis Longitudinal Study. Circulation 2008;118:2694–2701.
6 Lee M, Saver JL, Chang KH, Liao HW, Chang SC, Ovbiagele B: Impact of microalbuminuria on incident stroke: a meta-analysis. Stroke 2010;41:2625–2631.
7 Lee M, Saver JL, Chang KH, Liao HW, Chang SC, Ovbiagele B: Low glomerular filtration rate and risk of stroke: meta-analysis. BMJ 2010;341:c4249.
8 Etgen T, Chonchol M, Förstl H, Sander D: Chronic kidney disease and cognitive impairment: a systematic review and meta-analysis. Am J Nephrol 2012;35:474–482.
9 Vogels SC, Emmelot-Vonk MH, Verhaar HJ, Koek HD: The association of chronic kidney disease with brain lesions on MRI or CT: a systematic review. Maturitas 2012;71:331–336.

10 Yao H, Miwa Y, Takashima Y, Yahara K, Hashimoto M, Uchino A, Yuzuriha T, Sasaguri T: Chronic kidney disease and subclinical lacunar infarction are independently associated with frontal lobe dysfunction in community-dwelling elderly subjects: the Sefuri brain MRI study. Hypertens Res 2011;34: 1023–1028.
11 Matsuo S, Imai E, Horio M, Yasuda Y, Tomita K, Nitta K, Yamagata K, Tomino Y, Yokoyama H, Hishida A: Collaborators developing the Japanese equation for estimated GFR. Revised equations for estimated GFR from serum creatinine in Japan. Am J Kidney Dis 2009;53:982–992.
12 Chou CC, Lien LM, Chen WH, Wu MS, Lin SM, Chiu HC, Chiou HY, Bai CH: Adults with late stage 3 chronic kidney disease are at high risk for prevalent silent brain infarction: a population-based study. Stroke 2011;42: 2120–2125.
13 Sasaki M, Hirai T, Taoka T, Higano S, Wakabayashi C, Matsusue E, Ida M: Discriminating between silent cerebral infarction and deep white matter hyperintensity using combinations of three types of magnetic resonance images: a multicenter observer performance study. Neuroradiology 2008;50: 753–758.
14 O'Rourke MF, Safar ME: Relationship between aortic stiffening and microvascular disease in brain and kidney: cause and logic of therapy. Hypertension 2005;46:200–204.
15 Ito S, Nagasawa T, Abe M, Mori T: Strain vessel hypothesis: a viewpoint for linkage of albuminuria and cerebro-cardiovascular risk. Hypertens Res 2009;32:115–121.
16 Levey AS, Coresh J, Balk E, Kausz AT, Levin A, Steffes MW, Hogg RJ, Perrone RD, Lau J, Eknoyan G: National Kidney Foundation practice guidelines for chronic kidney disease: evaluation, classification, and stratification. Ann Intern Med 2003;139:137–147.
17 Khatri M, Wright CB, Nickolas TL, Yoshita M, Paik MC, Kranwinkel G, Sacco RL, DeCarli C: Chronic kidney disease is associated with white matter hyperintensity volume: the Northern Manhattan Study (NOMAS). Stroke 2007;38:3121–3126.
18 Ikram MA, Vernooij MW, Hofman A, Niessen WJ, van der Lugt A, Breteler MM: Kidney function is related to cerebral small vessel disease. Stroke 2008;39:55–61.
19 Seliger SL, Longstreth WT Jr, Katz R, Manolio T, Fried LF, Shlipak M, Stehman-Breen CO, Newman A, Sarnak M, Gillen DL, Bleyer A, Siscovick DS: Cystatin C and subclinical brain infarction. J Am Soc Nephrol 2005;16: 3721–3727.
20 Wada M, Nagasawa H, Iseki C, Takahashi Y, Sato H, Arawaka S, Kawanami T, Kurita K, Daimon M, Kato T: Cerebral small vessel disease and chronic kidney disease (CKD): results of a cross-sectional study in community-based Japanese elderly. J Neurol Sci 2008; 272:36–42.
21 Otani H, Kikuya M, Hara A, Terata S, Ohkubo T, Kondo T, Hirose T, Obara T, Metoki H, Inoue R, Asayama K, Kanno A, Terawaki H, Nakayama M, Totsune K, Hoshi H, Satoh H, Izumi S, Imai Y: Association of kidney dysfunction with silent lacunar infarcts and white matter hyperintensity in the general population: the Ohasama study. Cerebrovasc Dis 2010;30:43–50.
22 Kobayashi M, Hirawa N, Yatsu K, Kobayashi Y, Yamamoto Y, Saka S, Andoh D, Toya Y, Yasuda G, Umemura S: Relationship between silent brain infarction and chronic kidney disease. Nephrol Dial Transplant 2009;24: 201–207.
23 Shima H, Ishimura E, Naganuma T, Ichii M, Yamasaki T, Mori K, Nakatani T, Inaba M: Decreased kidney function is a significant factor associated with silent cerebral infarction and periventricular hyperintensities. Kidney Blood Press Res 2011;34:430–438.
24 Stinghen AE, Pecoits-Filho R: Vascular damage in kidney disease: beyond hypertension. Int J Hypertens 2011;2011:232683.
25 Shlipak MG, Fried LF, Crump C, Bleyer AJ, Manolio TA, Tracy RP, Furberg CD, Psaty BM: Elevations of inflammatory and procoagulant biomarkers in elderly persons with renal insufficiency. Circulation 2003;107:87–92.
26 Young JM, Terrin N, Wang X, Greene T, Beck GJ, Kusek JW, Collins AJ, Sarnak MJ, Menon V: Asymmetric dimethylarginine and mortality in stages 3 to 4 chronic kidney disease. Clin J Amm Soc Nephrol 2009;4:1115–1120.
27 Menon V, Li L, Wang X, Greene T, Balakrishnan V, Madero M, Pereira AA, Beck GJ, Kusek JW, Collins AJ, Levey AS, Sarnak MJ: Adiponectin and mortality in patients with chronic kidney disease. J Am Soc Nephrol 2006;17:2599–2606.

28 Kaisar OM, Johnson DW, Prins JB, Isbel N: The role of novel biomarkers of cardiovascular disease in chronic kidney disease: focus on adiponectin and leptin. Curr Cardiol Rev 2008;4:287–292.
29 Brady CB, Gaziano JM, Cxypoliski RA, Guarino PD, Kaufman JS, Warren SR, Hartigan P, Goldfarb DS, Jamison RL: Homocysteine lowering and cognition in CKD: the Veterans Affairs homocysteine study. Am J Kidney Dis 2009;54:440–449.
30 Mann JF, Sheridan P, McQueen MJ, Held C, Arnold JM, Fodor G, Yusuf S, Lonn EM, HOPE-2 Investigators: Homocysteine lowering with folic acid and B vitamins in people with chronic kidney disease – results of the renal Hope-2 study. Nephrol Dial Transplant 2008;23:645–653.

Hiroshi Yao, MD
Center for Emotional and Behavioral Disorders
National Hospital Organization Hizen Psychiatric Center
Mitsu 160, Yoshinogari, Kanzaki, Saga 842-0192 (Japan)
E-Mail hyao@hizen2.hosp.go.jp

Risk of Clinical and Subclinical Brain Damage in Kidney Disease

Toyoda K (ed): Brain, Stroke and Kidney.
Contrib Nephrol. Basel, Karger, 2013, vol 179, pp 35–41 (DOI: 10.1159/000346720)

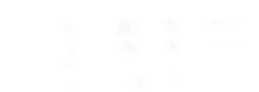

Carotid Atherosclerosis in Kidney Disease

Yoshihiro Kokubo

Department of Preventive Cardiology, National Cerebral and Cardiovascular Disease, Suita, Japan

Abstract

Recently, chronic kidney disease (CKD) has become a major public health problem and a risk factor for all-cause mortality, cardiovascular disease (CVD). To prevent cardiovascular disease as early as possible, subclinical studies for CKD are essential. Recently, carotid atherosclerosis has been evaluated by measurement of the intima-media thickness (IMT) of the carotid artery wall, which is a good predictor of incidence of CVD. In this manuscript, I reviewed subclinical studies on the relationship between the carotid atherosclerosis and kidney dysfunction in a general population. Cross-sectional studies for general populations have shown an inverse association of carotid IMT with renal function. In one large cross-sectional study in a US population, the cystatin C level had no independent association with carotid IMT. However, in cross-sectional studies for outpatients, a significant association was observed between the two in subjects with kidney dysfunction. The association between CKD and carotid IMT tends to be weaker in apparently healthy populations than in patients. A higher level of blood pressure decreases renal function, and a decreased GFR raises blood pressure. In other words, increases in blood pressure and decreases of renal function exacerbate each other. Therefore, an investigation of the incidence of CVD and subclinical analyses of both renal dysfunction and blood pressure categories is called for. The impact of high-normal blood pressure and hypertension on stenosis were more evident in subjects with CKD. Carotid atherosclerosis tended to be more severe in subjects with CKD and high blood pressure. These findings pointed to the importance of early detection of subjects with decreased renal function and the strict management of blood pressure in general populations.

Recently, in prospective follow-up studies for general populations, chronic kidney disease (CKD) has become a major public health problem and a risk factor for all-cause mortality, cardiovascular disease (CVD), and its subtypes such as stroke and myocardial infarction (MI) [1]. In end-stage renal disease, the cardiovascular disease mortality rate is more than 10 times as high as that in the general population [2]. Even at relatively high glomerular filtration rates (GFRs), renal dysfunction is an independent risk factor for incident CVD [1, 3]. In a large population sample from California (approximately 1.1 million people, mean age 52 years, 2.8 years of mean follow-up), compared with the estimated GFR (eGFR) ≥60 ml/min/1.73 m^2 group, the adjusted hazard ratios (95% CI) of all-cause mortality for eGFR = ranges of 45–59, 30–44, 15–29, and <15 ml/min/1.73 m^2 were 1.2 (1.1–1.2), 1.8 (1.7–1.9), 3.2 (3.1–3.4), and 5.9 (5.4–6.5). In an urban Japanese population sample, compared with the eGFR ≥90 ml/min/1.73 m^2 group, the hazard ratios (95% CIs) for the incidence of CVD and stroke were 1.8 (1.2–2.5) and 1.9 (1.3–3.0) in the eGFR = 50–59 ml/min/1.73 m^2 group and 2.5 (1.6–3.9) and 2.2 (1.2–4.1) in the eGFR <50 ml/min/1.73 m^2 group, respectively.

In order to prevent cardiovascular disease as early as possible, subclinical studies for CKD are essential. Recently, carotid atherosclerosis has been evaluated by measurement of the intima-media thickness (IMT) of the carotid artery wall, which is a good predictor of incidence of CVD [4]. It is important for persons with cardiovascular risk factors to be evaluated for carotid atherosclerosis before the onset of CVD. In this section, I would like to review subclinical studies on the association between carotid atherosclerosis and kidney dysfunction in a general population.

Kidney Dysfunction and Carotid Atherosclerosis

Table 1 shows a review of published articles on the association between kidney dysfunction and carotid atherosclerosis in various general populations. Among the three studies of Westerners, a cross-sectional study for Germany population showed that carotid IMT was increased by 0.02 mm (95% confidence intervals; 0.02 to 0.03 mm) in the 1st quartile, compared with the 4th quartile creatinine clearance [5]. In a study from Finland, carotid IMT was observed to be inversely associated with estimated GFR, although this study had a small sample size [6]. However, in a relatively large US population, the cystatin C level had no independent association with carotid IMT. Due to the wide age ranges in the US population, various cardiovascular risk factors are involved in carotid IMT. In Caucasian populations, kidney dysfunction may be weak but still a significant risk factor for carotid atherosclerosis nonetheless.

On the other hand, in Asian populations, CKD increases the risk of carotid atherosclerosis [7, 8]. A recent Japanese study has examined whether combinations of CKD with blood pressure category were associated with carotid arteriosclerosis. In hypertensive subjects, albuminuria and CKD were each associated with IMT (odds ratios = 1.85 and 1.79; 95% CIs = 1.13–3.03 and 1.09–2.94; p = 0.015 and 0.022, re-

Table 1. Review of the association between renal dysfunction and carotid atherosclerosis (general population)

Population	Number	Sex	Age, years	Study design	Results	Journal
Caucasian						
Germany	3,364	M/F	≥55	cross-sectional	compared with the 4th quartile creatinine clearance, IMT was increased by 0.02 (0.02–0.03) in the 1st quartile.	Am J Kidney Dis 2008;51:584–593
Finland	247 (M) 258 (F)	M/F	40–62	cross-sectional	IMT is inverse associated with eGFR	Nephrol Dial Transplant 2009;24:2767–2772
US	6,557	M/F	45–84	cross-sectional	cystatin C level had no independent association with carotid IMT	Am J Kidney Dis 2009;53:389–398
Asian						
China	1,046	MF	63±9	cross-sectional	IMT = 0.74±0.27 mm (eGFR >90), 0.82±0.30 (eGFR = 60–89), 0.94±0.38 (eGFR <60); p < 0.001	Am J Kidney Dis 2007;49:786–792
Japan	1,351	M	58±10	cross-sectional	hypertension+CKD(+): HR = 1.79 (1.09–2.94, p = 0.022); normotension+CKD(+): no association, albuminuria+CKD(+)+IFG or DM: increase risk of carotid early athero-screrosis, albuminuria+CKD(+)+IFG or DM: no association	Hypertens Res 2007;30:1035–1041

IFG = Impaired fasting glucose; DM = diabetes mellitus; HR = hazard ratio.

spectively), but neither was associated with carotid IMT in subjects with normotension. In addition, combination of albuminuria and CKD was significantly associated with IMT in subjects with impaired fasting glucose (fasting plasma glucose levels ≥110 mg/dl or current use of antidiabetic medication), but not in those without. In order to evaluate the association between CKD and IMT, other cardiovascular risk factors, that is blood pressure should be also considered.

Table 2 summarizes the previous published articles on the association between kidney dysfunction and carotid atherosclerosis in patients. In Caucasian outpatients, a significant association was observed in subjects with kidney dysfunction [9–12]. In Chinese predialysis patients, carotid IMT shows statistically significant increases according to the stage of CKD [13]. Overall, the association between CKD and carotid IMT tend to be weaker in apparently healthy populations than in patients. Therefore, to detect the association between kidney dysfunction and carotid atherosclerosis, present illnesses should be considered, especially cardiovascular disease, i.e., higher blood pressure. The total population-attributable fractions of higher blood pressure for cardiovascular disease have been estimated as approximately 50% in men and 30% in women [14].

Table 2. Review of the association between renal dysfunction and carotid atherosclerosis (outpatients)

Population	Subjects	Number	Sex	Age, years	Study design	Results	Journal
Caucasian							
UK	cases, outpatients plasma creatinine >1.4 mg/dl; control, 13 healthy normotensive	cases/ control: 114/13	MF	66 (55–71)	cross-sectional	common carotid artery-IMT: cases, 0.59±0.22 mm; control, 0.44±0.08 mm; p = 0.0012	Am J Kidney Dis 2005;46:856–862
France	CKD/hypertension /normotension patients	273	MF	58±15/ 59± 11/ 56±6	cross-sectional	IMT: no association; internal diastolic diameter = 6.3±1.1/ 5.8±0.7/5.5±0.6 (p < 0.001)	Kidney Int 2006;69:350–357
Australia	chronic renal failure patients	159:159	MF	64±8	case-control	0.89±0.17 vs. 0.73±0.13 mm, p < 0.05	Clin Exp Pharmacol Physiol 2000;27:639–641
Brazil	outpatients	122	MF	55±11	cross-sectional	IMT = 0.62±0.19 (eGFR <60) vs. 0.53±0.10 mm (eGFR >60); p = 0.030	Nephron Clin Pract 2010;115: c189–194
Asian							
China	predialysis CKD patients	227	MF	56±16	cross-sectional	0.64±0.18 (CKD I-II), 0.74±0.25 (CKD III), 0.81±0.25 (CKD IV), 0.86±0.20 (CKD V), p < 0.01	Eur J Int Med 2012;23:539–544

IFG = Impaired fasting glucose; DM = diabetes mellitus; HR = hazard ratio.

Subclinical Organ Damage

According to the 2007 European Society of Cardiology/European Society of Hypertension (ESC/ESH) Guidelines for the management of arterial hypertension [15] and the Japanese Society of Hypertension Guidelines for the Management of Hypertension (JSH 2009) [16], the risk of CVD was stratified by blood pressure categories and cardiovascular risk factors. The strata of the 2007 ESC/ESH Guideline consist of the first stratum (no risk factors), the second stratum (1–2 risk factors), the third stratum (3 or more risk factors, metabolic syndrome, or subclinical organ damage), and the fourth stratum. CKD is categorized in third stratum as subclinical organ damage (the third stratum), based on slight increases in plasma creatinine (men 1.3–1.5 mg/dl; women 1.2–1.4 mg/dl), microalbuminuria (30–300 mg), and low estimated glomerular filtration rate by the MDRD formula (<60 ml/min/1.73 m^2) or creatinine clearance by the Cockroft Gault formula (<60 ml/min). According to the 2007 ESC/ESH Guideline, the blood pressure category should be optimal blood pressure in order to prevent CVD from contributing to subclinical kidney damage.

In an urban cohort, compared with optimal blood pressure subjects without CKD, the normal blood pressure, high-normal blood pressure, and hypertensive subjects without CKD showed increased risks of CVD, whereas the impact of each blood pressure category on CVD was more evident in subjects with CKD, especially in men (p for interaction = 0.04) [3]. Results of stroke were similar (p for interaction = 0.03 in men).

Recently, in a prospective cohort study, CKD in the high-normal blood pressure category at the baseline survey has been a risk factor for incident hypertension (multivariable-adjusted hazard ratio = 1.41) [17]. In an urban population cohort of Nagoya, Japan, the adjusted hazard ratio (95% CI) of incident hypertension in the highest tertile of GFR (4.4–76.1 ml/min/1.73 m^2) was 1.40 (1.26–1.57) compared with the first tertile [18]. A reduction in GFR of 10 ml/min/1.73 m^2 was associated with an 11% increase in risk for incident hypertension. In other studies, renal dysfunction has been associated with increased levels of inflammatory factors [19, 20], abnormal apolipoprotein levels [19], elevated plasma homocysteine [19], enhanced coagulability [20], anemia, left ventricular hypertrophy, increased arterial calcification, endothelial dysfunction and arterial stiffness [21]. These factors may contribute to elevated blood pressure.

On the other hand, The Multiple Risk Factor Intervention Trial study, one of the coronary heart disease prevention trials recommended to the National Heart and Lung Institute in US, showed that elevations of blood pressure are a strong independent risk factor for end-stage renal disease [22]. Compared with optimal blood pressure, hypertension is a risk factor for end-stage renal disease, with adjusted relative risks (95% CIs) for stages 1–4 hypertension of 3.1 (2.3–4.3), 6.0 (4.3–8.4), 11.2 (7.7–16.2) and 22.1 (14.2–34.3), respectively. A higher level of blood pressure decreases renal function [22], and a decreased GFR raises blood pressure. In other words, increases in blood pressure and decreases of renal function exacerbate each other.

Recently, the Suita Study has shown that CKD is independently associated with carotid atherosclerosis, especially in GFR <50 ml/min/1.73 m^2 (odds ratio = 1.91; 95% CI = 1.16–3.14) in a general urban population (1,602 men and 1,844 women) [23]. The impact of high-normal blood pressure and hypertension on stenosis were more evident in subjects with CKD (high-normal blood pressure: odds ratios (95% CIs) = 1.58 (1.08–2.31) and 2.74 (1.63–4.61); hypertension: odds ratios = 1.94 (1.36–2.77) and 2.36 (1.49–3.73) in non-CKD and CKD groups, respectively). Carotid atherosclerosis tended to be more severe in subjects with CKD and high blood pressure. This study suggests the importance of early detection of subjects with decreased renal function and the strict management of blood pressure in the general population.

Conclusions

This review found that the association between renal function and carotid IMT tends to be weaker in general populations than that in outpatients. Increases in blood pressure and decreases of renal function exacerbate each other. A cross-sectional study in an urban population has shown that the impact of high-normal blood pressure and hypertension on stenosis were more evident in subjects with CKD. These findings stress the importance of early detection of subjects with decreased renal function and the strict management of blood pressure in general populations in order to prevent CVD in early stage. Additional studies are required to assess whether lowering of eGFR can actually increase the risk of carotid atherosclerosis according to blood pressure category in cohort study.

Acknowledgement

The present study was supported by the Intramural Research Fund of the National Cerebral and Cardiovascular Center (22–4–5) and by a grant (No. 23390178) from the Ministry of Education, Science, and Culture of Japan.

References

1 Go AS, Chertow GM, Fan D, McCulloch CE, Hsu CY: Chronic kidney disease and the risks of death, cardiovascular events, and hospitalization. N Engl J Med 2004;351:1296–1305.
2 USRDS: The United States renal data system. Am J Kidney Dis 2003;42:1–230.
3 Kokubo Y, Nakamura S, Okamura T, Yoshimasa Y, Makino H, Watanabe M, et al: Relationship between blood pressure category and incidence of stroke and myocardial infarction in an urban Japanese population with and without chronic kidney disease: the Suita study. Stroke 2009;40:2674–2679.
4 Kokubo Y, Toyoda K, Watanabe M, Ono Y, Miyamoto Y, Nagatsuka K: Impact of carotid plaque on the risk of stroke and ischemic heart disease in a Japanese urban population: the Suita study. Cerebrovasc Dis 2011;31(suppl 2):7.
5 Desbien AM, Chonchol M, Gnahn H, Sander D: Kidney function and progression of carotid intima-media thickness in a community study. Am J Kidney Dis 2008;51:584–593.
6 Kastarinen H, Ukkola O, Kesaniemi YA: Glomerular filtration rate is related to carotid intima-media thickness in middle-aged adults. Nephrol Dial Transplant 2009;24:2767–2772.
7 Zhang L, Zhao F, Yang Y, Qi L, Zhang B, Wang F, et al: Association between carotid artery intima-media thickness and early-stage CKD in a Chinese population. Am J Kidney Dis 2007;49:786–792.
8 Ishizaka N, Ishizaka Y, Toda E, Koike K, Seki G, Nagai R, et al: Association between chronic kidney disease and carotid intima-media thickening in individuals with hypertension and impaired glucose metabolism. Hypertens Res 2007;30:1035–1041.
9 Lemos MM, Jancikic AD, Sanches FM, Christofalo DM, Ajzen SA, Carvalho AB, et al: Intima-media thickness is associated with inflammation and traditional cardiovascular risk factors in non-dialysis-dependent patients with chronic kidney disease. Nephron Clin Pract 2010;115:c189–c194.

10 Zoungas S, Ristevski S, Lightfoot P, Liang YL, Branley P, Shiel LM, et al: Carotid artery intima-medial thickness is increased in chronic renal failure. Clin Exp Pharmacol Physiol 2000;27:639–641.
11 Briet M, Bozec E, Laurent S, Fassot C, London GM, Jacquot C, et al: Arterial stiffness and enlargement in mild-to-moderate chronic kidney disease. Kidney Int 2006;69:350–357.
12 Preston E, Ellis MR, Kulinskaya E, Davies AH, Brown EA: Association between carotid artery intima-media thickness and cardiovascular risk factors in CKD. Am J Kidney Dis 2005;46:856–862.
13 Zhou W, Ni Z, Yu Z, Shi B, Wang Q: Brain natriuretic peptide is related to carotid plaques and predicts atherosclerosis in predialysis patients with chronic kidney disease. Eur J Int Med 2012;23:539–544.
14 Kokubo Y, Kamide K, Okamura T, Watanabe M, Higashiyama A, Kawanishi K, et al: Impact of high-normal blood pressure on the risk of cardiovascular disease in a Japanese urban cohort: the Suita study. Hypertension 2008;52: 652–659.
15 Mancia G, De Backer G, Dominiczak A, Cifkova R, Fagard R, Germano G, et al: 2007 guidelines for the management of arterial hypertension. The task force for the management of arterial hypertension of the European Society of Hypertension (ESH) and of the European Society of Cardiology (ESC). J Hypertens 2007;25:1105–1187.
16 Ogihara T, Kikuchi K, Matsuoka H, Fujita T, Higaki J, Horiuchi M, et al: The Japanese Society of Hypertension guidelines for the management of hypertension (JSH 2009). Hypertens Res 2009;32:3–107.
17 Kokubo Y, Nakamura S, Watanabe M, Kamide K, Kawano Y, Kawanishi K, et al: Cardiovascular risk factors associated with incident hypertension according to blood pressure categories in non-hypertensive population in the Suita Study: an urban cohort study. Hypertension 2011;58:e100.
18 Takase H, Dohi Y, Toriyama T, Okado T, Tanaka S, Sonoda H, et al: Evaluation of risk for incident hypertension using glomerular filtration rate in the normotensive general population. J Hypertens 2012;30:505–512.
19 Muntner P, Hamm LL, Kusek JW, Chen J, Whelton PK, He J: The prevalence of nontraditional risk factors for coronary heart disease in patients with chronic kidney disease. Ann Intern Med 2004;140:9–17.
20 Shlipak MG, Fried LF, Crump C, Bleyer AJ, Manolio TA, Tracy RP, et al: Elevations of inflammatory and procoagulant biomarkers in elderly persons with renal insufficiency. Circulation 2003;107:87–92.
21 Feldman HI, Appel LJ, Chertow GM, Cifelli D, Cizman B, Daugirdas J, et al: The chronic renal insufficiency cohort (CRIC) study: Design and methods. J Am Soc Nephrol 2003; 14:S148–S153.
22 Klag MJ, Whelton PK, Randall BL, Neaton JD, Brancati FL, Ford CE, et al: Blood pressure and end-stage renal disease in men. N Engl J Med 1996;334:13–18.
23 Ohara T, Kokubo Y, Toyoda K, Koga M, Nagatsuka K, Nakamura S, et al: The impact of chronic kidney disease on carotid atherosclerosis in a general Japanese urban population: the Suita study. Stroke 2012;43:A2642.

Yoshihiro Kokubo, MD, PhD, FAHA, FACC, FESC
Department of Preventive Cardiology
National Cerebral and Cardiovascular Center
5-7-1, Fujishiro-dai, Suita, Osaka, 565-8565 (Japan)
E-Mail ykokubo@hsp.ncvc.go.jp

Risk of Clinical and Subclinical Brain Damage in Kidney Disease

Toyoda K (ed): Brain, Stroke and Kidney.
Contrib Nephrol. Basel, Karger, 2013, vol 179, pp 42–57 (DOI: 10.1159/000346722)

Kidney Disease and Cognitive Function

Merrill F. Elias[a] · Gregory A. Dore[b] · Adam Davey[c]

[a]Department of Psychology and Graduate School of Biomedical Sciences and [b]Department of Psychology, The University of Maine, Orono, Me., and [c]Department of Public Health, Temple University, Philadelphia, Pa., USA

Abstract

We provide a brief review of research on chronic kidney disease and cognitive performance, including dementia. We touch briefly on the literature relating end-stage-renal disease to cognitive function, but focus on studies of modest and moderate forms of chronic kidney disease (CKD) that precede dialysis and transplantation. We summarize previous reviews dealing with case control studies of patients but more fully examine community-based studies with large samples and necessary controls for demographic risk factors, cardiovascular variables, and other confounds such as depression. In addition we suggest potential biological and social-psychological mediators between CKD and cognition. Studies follow in two categories of design: (1) cross-sectional studies, and (2) longitudinal studies. In each, CKD is related to a wide range of deficits in cognitive functioning including verbal and visual memory and organization, and components of executive functioning and fluid intellect. In general, prior to the need to treat with hemodialysis (HD) or kidney transplant (KT), magnitude of effect with relation to CKD and function are small or modest in persons free from acute stroke and dementia. However, HD and KT can result in major impairment. We discuss needed controls, the greater demand on controls after the start of HD and KT, and suggest that mechanisms intervening relations between hypertension, or diabetes, and cognitive performance may be similar to those intervening between hypertension and cognitive performance and the hypertension and diabetes literature on cognition provides a good model for the study of early stage kidney disease and cognitive ability. We posit that the mechanisms linking CKD and cognition may be similar to those linking hypertension or diabetes to cognition. We identify the need for more studies with multiple cognitive test batteries, measures of every-day cognitive abilities relevant to patient understanding of the disease and treatments, and more studies with prevalent and incident dementia outcomes. Descriptors: kidney disease, chronic kidney disease, cognitive function, dementia and cardiovascular risk factors.

Table 1. Common predictor variables in studies of renal disease and cognitive performance

Predictor	Metric or type of measurement	Type of variable
Uremic patient[1] vs. controls	diagnostic criteria	categorical
eGFR[2]	ml/min/1.73 m^2 body surface	categorical[4] or continuous
Serum creatinine (sCR)	mg/dl or μmol/l	continuous[5]
Stage of kidney disease[3]	standard diagnostic criteria	categorical

[1] Uremia defined as the accumulation of urinary waste products in the urine or the constellation of signs and symptoms indicating kidney disease or failure.
[2] eGFR can be estimated via different formulae: modification of diet in renal disease (MDRD) study equation; chronic kidney disease epidemiology collaboration (CKD-EPI) equation; Mayo Clinic Quadratic equation.
[3] See reference 5 for definitions and criteria.
[4] Studies often use eGFR ≥60 (ml/min/1.73 m^2) versus <60, or, for example, normal (≥90); mildly decreased (60 to 89); moderate CKD (30–59), severe CKD (15 to 29) and kidney failure (<15), or clinical criteria, tertiles, quartiles, quintiles etc.
[5] Continuously distributed such as eGFR in units (ml/min/1.73 m^2) or sCR in units (1 mg/dl) expressed as 1/sCR due to skew [e.g. 26].

A new case of dementia occurs every 4 seconds worldwide, which is equivalent to 7.7 million cases each year, and mild cognitive impairment is even more prevalent [1]. Chronic kidney disease (CKD) is a risk factor (RF) for dementia and cognitive decline [2, 3–5]. Cognitive impairment detracts from quality of life and is a risk factor for dialysis-related mortality [6]. In this brief review we summarize the literature on CKD in relation to cognitive function, discuss intervening mechanisms, and comment on some methodological issues, but refer the reader to other reviews of the many studies comparing treatments such as hemodialysis (HD), peritoneal dialysis (PD) and transplantation. We emphasize a pretreatment stage of CKD, but include studies examining modest to severe CKD.

Renal Functioning Predictors of Cognitive Function

Renal disease is well-defined in previous reviews [2, 3, 5, 7]. Table 1 summarizes commonly used predictor variables in cognitive studies and the measurement metrics used to define them. Common predictors are estimated glomerular filtration rate (eGFR), serum creatinine (sCR) and far less commonly stages of renal disease [2] involving measures such a proteinuria, biopsy or structural imaging.

Cognitive Outcomes in Renal Studies

A previous review provides a list of tests commonly used in the renal literature [3] and other reviews illustrate how multiple tests should be used where the goal is to infer the locus of brain impairment from one or more specific cognitive deficits [8, 9]. Studies designed to examine which abilities do and do not relate to a disease must examine a wide range of different abilities [8, 9]. Definitions of terms used in the psychometric literature are given in table 2. Outcome variables can be dichotomous (i.e. dementia, impairment, deficit), ordinal categories of performance level, or continuously distributed test scores representing performance level. We use the term cognitive impairment only if this cognitive status has been established by clinical criteria, i.e. neuropsychological (NP) evaluation and/or normative data. The term deficit is used as a comparative term indicating a lower average level of performance relative to a reference group or groups. The term decline is only used for longitudinal change in performance.

Overview: End-Stage Renal Disease and Treatment

We refer the reader to previous reviews [2, 3, 5] for a summary of this literature. However, it is important to note that an estimated 70% of HD patients over age 55 exhibit moderate-to-severe cognitive impairment [5] with a similar prevalence for PD patients [10]. Griva et al. [6] reported that two-thirds of a community-dwelling sample of 145 PD, home dialysis and in-center HD patients in London, UK, suffered from what the authors defined as mild or moderate cognitive impairment: 1.00–1.99 and 2–2.99 SD below the mean, respectively. We agree with Murray and Knopman [5] that performance 2.00 SD below the mean (2% of the population fall here) is not moderate, but is reflective of clinically significant cognitive dysfunction. Comprehensive reviews of this literature indicate that HD, PD and transplantation are associated with wide ranging deficits in attention, memory, speed of performance, and components of executive functioning (EF) [5], although it is clear that adverse cognitive outcomes are attenuated when cognitive testing is timed properly in relation to dialysis treatment [2].

There have been few studies of practical everyday cognitive tasks and kidney disease. Numeracy skills are critical to advance planning necessary to comply with treatment regimens and disease understanding [11]. Numeracy refers to the degree that one can apply statistical, graphical and numerical skills in such a way as to effectively understand and comply with health information [11]. Abdel-Kader et al. [11] found that the majority of 187 end-stage renal disease

Table 2. Definitions of terms used in this review

Term	Definition
Construct	The theoretical mental process that tests attempt to measure or index.
Decline	Change in performance level from better to worse over time.
Deficit	A relative decrement in performance that does not rise to the level of impairment, e.g. mean level of performance in a group is lower than mean level of performance in another group, but individual differences in performance may overlap among groups.
Dementia	A progressive cognitive impairment characterized by decline in memory ability and impairment in one or more other cognitive domains, e.g., language, orientation, reasoning, attention and EF. Represents a decline from a previous level of functioning and interferes with activities of daily living and independence. AD is the most common form and a major risk factor is amnestic MCI.
Domain	A composite set of skills measured (indexed) by more than one test of specific ability as may be identified by factor analysis.
Everyday ability	A test that measures real-life activities such as map reading, check balancing, following directions, organizing medications.
Executive function	The ability to anticipate, plan and organize and to reject old inappropriate responses for new appropriate responses when confronted with a new problem. Difficult to separate from fluid intelligence and often and erroneously used as isomorphic with frontal lobe function, although frontal lobe damage is associated with poorer EF.
Fluid intelligence	Ability with regard to dealing with new and novel tasks as opposed to crystallized (verbal intelligence) ability, often with demands on speed of performance. Many reviews of the literature have emphasized the extreme difficulty of separating fluid intelligence from EF given their significant overlap in abilities measured [9]
Global ability	Overall ability which is the synergistic combination of specific abilities, e.g. overall score on an intelligence test.
Impairment	Poor performance reaching a clinically important level of deficit as defined by neuropsychological assessment and/or normative data.
Impurity	Failure of a test to measure only abilities it was designed to measure.
Level of performance	An average or median level of performance based on the entire distribution of test scores or normative data.
Mental status	Ability measured by screening measures such as the Mini Mental Status Examination (MMSE), often described as a test of global ability but lacking in sensitivity and specificity relative to intelligence test measures.
Mild cognitive impairment	Mild cognitive impairment is a level of performance that indicates decline from a previous level of performance and impairment by clinical/normative criteria, but does not rise to the level of dementia. Individuals with mild cognitive impairment typically remain in the community and do not necessarily exhibit general intellectual decline. There are at least 30 different formal clinical definitions in the literature.

Table 2. Continued

Term	Definition
Short form	A shorter form of a test designed to retain validity and reliability but normally looses both to some extent.
Specific ability	Ability in a relatively narrow range of specialized functioning as opposed to global cognitive ability or general intelligence.
Vascular dementia (VaD)	Memory decline may be present but not necessarily predominant and other cognitive domains are affected early in the disease process and in the MCI that precedes it. Progress of VaD is more varied over time than is the progress of AD and a history of CVD risk factors and events are common. AD has a vascular component and mixed dementias are common.

(ESRD) patients (mean age = 52 years) exhibited low numeric efficiency on a 3-item scale. Grubbs et al. [12] reported a 32.3% prevalence of inadequate health care literacy in a sample of 62 dialysis patients. Gelb and colleagues [13], in a study of 108 kidney transplant recipients, reported that lower levels of performance on everyday problem-solving tests and number of depressive symptoms were associated with poor medication adherence, but found no association with multiple NP measures and adherence. These studies were not prospective and thus the direction of these associations needs to be defined in future studies.

In summary, the history of cognitive deficit and impairment begins prior to the transition to ESRD [5]. Once ESRD status has been reached and dialysis has begun, the demands on design and control become increasingly complex and thus the early or pre-treatment stages of CKD provide an important window of investigation.

Cross-Sectional Community-Based Studies

We have chosen to focus on the community-based studies given the very much larger samples, statistical adjustment for CVD and absence of sample bias introduced by multiple exclusions in order control for differences in health factors among uremic samples, healthy controls and patient groups.

Table 5 summarizes methodological detail and results for the community-based studies which began to appear in 2005. Earlier investigations emphasized case-control type studies that compared uremic patients to other diagnostic groups, e.g. medical and psychiatric patients or healthy controls [2]. A major review of this case-control literature [2] indicates that uremic patients, compared to general medical and psychiatric groups, performed better on measures of motor speed, auditory alertness and crystallized intelligence and performed more poorly on measures of cognitive flexibility and other components of EF, verbal memory and learning, visual attention and fluid intelligence. In 3 of the case-control studies reviewed by Koushik et al. [2], levels of performance were not below average when compared to normative data. In some case-control studies exclusion for health factors were extensive [e.g.14], but often the major controls were for age, education, and sex [2].

In each of the community-based studies (table 3) there were controls (exclusion or adjustment) for demographic variables, CVD risk factors, or health factors, and other confounders. Estimated eGFR levels <60 versus ≥60 were associated with deficits in global cognitive performance. Studies prior to 2009 reported that higher levels of eGFR were associated with deficits in language, memory, components of EF [15, 16], learning and concentration [15], visual attention [15], psychomotor efficiency and processing speed [17], and global impairment on a telephone interview scale [18]. While sample sizes were impressive, the cognitive batteries were limited, sometimes involving only one or a few tests.

To address this issue, Elias et al. [19] using the Maine Syracuse Longitudinal Study (MSLS), employed 923 dementia-free community-dwelling individuals and 19 widely-used clinical cognitive tests in a factor analysis leading to the identification of the following outcome variables: (1) a global composite test score, (2) four composite scores or factors: visual-spatial organization and memory, scanning and tracking (a component of executive function), verbal memory, and working memory, and (3) a single measure of abstract reasoning (WAIS similarities) which loaded with approximately equal strength on each composite. Persons undergoing dialysis (n = 4) and/or diagnosed with dementia (n = 9) were excluded. For an analysis adjusting for demographic factors, CVD, and acute stroke, higher sCR values were associated with lower levels of performance for global performance, verbal episodic memory and scanning and tracking. For example increments in creatinine of 2 mg/dl were associated with a decrement of 0.12 SD in performance level. Moreover, the odds ratios (ORs) associated with poor global performance (defined as the lowest quartile of the distribution of test scores) were OR = 2.27 with control for age, sex, education, and race and OR = 1.97 with additional adjustment for CVD and stroke.

In summary, community-based, large sample, cross-sectional studies support the generalization that mild and modest kidney disease is related to modest deficits in multiple cognitive abilities. As in the hypertension literature, crystallized intellect appears to be spared in studies of dementia-free samples [19]. The limitation of each of these studies is that they were cross-sectional and only two studies specifically reported excluding of dialysis patients [19, 20] or those with eGFR <30 [15].

Table 3. Community-based studies published after 2004 arranged by date of publication

Authors	Design	Outcomes	Control or adjustment	Summary of Findings
Kurella et al. [16] (2005)	1,105 community-dwelling postmenopausal women (<80 years) with established coronary artery disease (no hysterectomy) enrolled in the Estrogen/Progestin Replacement Study. CKD estimated using eGFR as mild (45–59), moderate (30–44) and severe (eGFR <30); eGFR ≥60 was the reference group.	Multiple tests including 3MS, Trail Making Part B, Boston Naming, Verbal Fluency, Word List Memory and Recall.	Adjustment for age, race, education, lifestyle factors, stroke, diabetes, and other variables related to kidney disease.	eGFR was associated with deficits in global cognition, executive function, language, and memory (15–25% increment in risk for deficit per 10 ml/min/1.73 m^2 decrement in eGFR.
Hailpern et al. [15] (2007) Level expressed as quartiles, referent group is quartile with the poorest performance.	Younger, healthy and ethnically diverse community-based adults recruited from the NHANES III (age range 20–59; N range 4,721 to 4,865 depending on the test used). Moderate CKD was defined as eGFR 30 to 59 with eGFR >60 as the reference group.	Simple visual-motor reaction time, visual attention and learning and concentration tests.	Ordinal regression analysis, adjustment for demographic variables and self-reported health variables. Diabetes excluded in sensitivity analyses.	Moderate CKD was associated with poorer learning and concentration (OR = 2.4) and visual attention (OR = 2.7) when adjusted for age, gender, education, race, and self-reported general health and other variables related to CKD.
Jassal et al. [17] (2008) Performance level (test scores).	99 uremic patients (mean age 65, with 50% >65 years) with stage 3–5 kidney disease on optimized medical treatment at a predialysis clinic. Renal function defined as eGFR calculated as a continuously distributed variable.	Multiple cognitive tests with composite scores measuring three domains : attention and working memory; psychomotor efficiency and processing speed; learning efficiency.	Adjustment for age, education and sex, comorbid diseases, hemoglobin, PTH, and number of neurodepressor drugs. antidepression medication, parathyroid diseases. Sensitivity analysis with ESPS. Exclusions: head injury, learning disabilities, history of acute stroke and TIA, and depressed mood.	Renal function (eGFR) was related to poorer performance on test of psychomotor efficiency and processing speed with statistical adjustment for covariates, but was not associated with performance scores for attention and working memory or learning ability.
Kurella Tamura et al. [18] (2008)	23,405 community-dwelling participants (>44 years) from the REGARDS Study. CKD defined as <60. eGFR in 10-ml/min/1.73 m^2 increments.	A six item telephone screening test with cognitive impairment (sic. deficit) defined as a score of <4.	Excluded eGFR <10. Adjusted for age, education, sex, race, recruitment location, CVD and CVD risk factors.	CKD <60 was associated with higher risk of cognitive deficit (OR = 1.23). Each 1-ml/min 1.73 m^2 was associated with an increment in cognitive impairment (OR = 1.11).

Table 3. Continued

Authors	Design	Outcomes	Control or adjustment	Summary of Findings
Elias et al. [19][1] (2009) Performance decrement defined as the lowest quartile and also performance level.	923 community dwelling participants (>40 years of age); comparisons between eGFR >60 and ≤60; increment in sCR from 1 to 2 mg/dl, and 1/sCR as a continuously distributed variable.	Based on 19 tests submitted to factor analysis. Composite scores were formed for verbal episodic memory (VEM), visual-spatial memory and organization, (VSOM) scanning and tracking (ST), working memory (WM), and a global composite of all scores.	Adjusted for age, education, sex, race, diabetes, systolic blood pressure, BMI, smoking, HDL and stroke and other risk factors in sensitivity analyses. Exclusions: dialysis, dementia, <40 years of age.	Comparisons of persons with eGFR ≥60 with eGFR <60 indicated decrement for the latter group for the global composite, OR = 1.25, VSOM, OR = 1.88), and ST (components of EF), OR = 1.56. Same associations for performance level outcomes. Higher levels of creatinine were associated with lower levels of performance on the global composite, WM, and ST.

Longitudinal Studies

Longitudinal studies of community-based samples after 2004 are summarized in table 4. These studies measure change in cognitive functioning over time. Studies are arranged by outcomes: (1) level of cognitive performance, (2) binary levels of performance where decline in performance is based on poor performance at follow-up defined arbitrarily or in terms of normative data, and (3) binary or gradations of certainty with regard to probable dementia. The first two categories are important to the third because lower cognitive performance in persons free from acute stroke and dementia is a risk factor for dementia [21]. The studies cited have relatively good controls as defined by adjustment for age, sex, education, and race, where relevant, and extended models which consider health variables, cardiovascular risk factors or events (e.g. stroke). Table 5 provides a check-list summary of results for papers summarized in table 4. Each of the studies [20, 22–28] reported that baseline levels for at least one predictor was related to cognitive decline, impairment or dementia, except for Slinin et al. [29] who obtained negative results with adjustment for age. Davey et al. [4] with the smallest longitudinal sample (n = 590), but with a comprehensive cognitive test battery, did not find longitudinal change in cognitive performance from base-

Table 4. Longitudinal studies of relations between kidney function and cognitive function organized by type of outcome (see italics): levels, impairment, dementia

Authors, outcome and time to follow-up	Predictor(s)	Controls: adjustments or exclusions
Buchman et al. [22] (2009) *Decline* in performance over 3.4 years.	Continuous eGFR (MDRD) at baseline and trichotomized impaired kidney function at baseline defined as <45, >45 to <60, >60.	eGFR at baseline, age, sex, education, BMI, hemoglobin, physical activity, social activity, vascular risk factors, vascular diseases, depressive symptoms. Exclusions: dementia.
Jassal et al. [24] (2010) Annual *decline* in performance level over mean follow-up of 6.6 years.	eGFR categorized as ≥60 or <60 and albuminuria (ACR ≥30 mg/g) versus no albuminuria.	Stratified by sex. Covariates: age, SBP, HbA1C, education, strenuous exercise, alcohol consumption, current estrogen for women, eGFR, depressed mood, antihypertensive meds, lipid-lowering meds, Exclusions: <50 years of age, stroke.
Wang et al. [28] (2010) *Decline* in performance over 4 years. (yes/no) in relation to baseline eGFR.	Categories of eGFR: ≥90 (reference), 60--89, 30–59; continuous eGFR in secondary analyses; albuminuria defined as ≥25 mg/g for males and ≥17 mg/g for females.	Basic: age, sex, education, BMI Additional: SBP, diabetes, urinary ACR. Exclusions: stroke.
Davey et al. [4] *Decline* in level of performance (over 4–5 years).	Continuously distributed eGFR and 1/sCR and change in eGFR baseline to follow-up.	Basic controls: age, education, sex race/ethnicity, eGFR at baseline. Additional controls: diabetes, depressed mood, alcohol consumption, diabetes and hypertension, APOE genotype, smoking, and cardiovascular disease. Exclusions, stroke at baseline dementia and renal dialysis.
Kurella et al. [25] (2005) *Incident impairment* (yes/no) with follow-up at 2 and 4 years.	Categories of eGFR: ≥60 (reference), 45–59, <45. Also used estimated creatinine clearance (Cockroft-Gault) and gender-specific creatinine cut-points (top 1 and 10% of distributions).	Basic: age, race, gender, education Additional: baseline CVD, diabetes, BP, lipids, inflammatory markers, hematocrit concentration, incident stroke Exclusions: baseline cognitive impairment; ADL difficulties; life-threatening illness; intention of moving before follow-up.
Slinin et al. [29] (2008) *Incident impairment* (yes/no) in follow-up 4.6 years.	eGFR (MDRD) categories, ≥60: 45–59 (mild CKD), <45 (moderate CKD).	Basic: age, education, race Additional: health status, IADL impairments, alcohol use, diabetes, hypertension, stroke, CVD, BMI, PAD Exclusions: unable to walk; bilateral hip replacement; severe medical conditions, dialysis excluded in secondary analyses.
Etgen et al. [20] (2009) *Incident impairment* over 2 years (yes/no) from in relation to baseline eGFR.	Baseline normal (>60) mild (45–59), and moderate-to-severe (<45) CKD based on eGFR (Cockroft-Gault standardized for body surface area).	Basic: age, sex Additional: depression, physical activity, alcohol, diabetes, IHD/stroke, hyperlipidemia, hypertension, smoking Exclusions: cognitive impairment at baseline; CKD at baseline in secondary analyses.

Sample	Cognitive tests or diagnostic category	Major statistically significant findings[1]
886 community-dwelling participants (mean age = 80.6) from the Rush Memory and Aging Project who participated in both baseline and follow-up analyses.	5 subscale composites and a global composite derived from 19 individual measures. Subscales were: episodic memory, semantic memory, working memory, perceptual speed, visuospatial abilities.	Lower eGFR and impaired kidney function associated with rate of decline in global composite, episodic memory, semantic memory, and working memory.
759 community dwelling men and women (mean age = 74.9 years) at baseline who returned for repeat testing.	MMSE, Trails B, and Animals Naming Category Fluency test performance levels, both continuous and using cut points.	For men but not women, baseline albuminuria, but not eGFR, was associated with decline in MMSE and category fluency scores with adjustment for all covariates.
1,243 community-based Chinese participants (≥40 years of age) with an eGFR >30; and 66 cases of during a 4-year follow-up.	A fall in MMSE of ≥2 points from baseline was defined as cognitive decline.	Relative to the reference group, risk of decline was higher for those with eGFR of 30–59.
590 Maine-Syracuse Longitudinal Study participants who participated at baseline and follow-up.	Decline in performance level for abstract reasoning and 4 major domains of functioning based on factor analysis of 19 separate test scores.	Baseline levels of eGFR and 1/sCR were unrelated to longitudinal change but change in renal function (eGFR) longitudinally was associated with change in cognitive performance for the global composite, verbal memory composite, and Similarities with all controls employed.
2,406 elderly persons in the Health ABC Study (mean age = 74 years).	Modified Mini-Mental State Exam (3MS) with incident 'impairment' defined as 3MS <80 or decline in 3MS >5 at either follow-up exam.	eGFR levels <60 were associated with greater odds of cognitive impairment, with adjustment for the full model. Creatinine levels in the top 10 and 1% were associated with higher odds of cognitive impairment, with adjustment for the basic model.
3,722 community-based men (≥65 years) from the Osteoporotic Fractures in Men Study who provided baseline and follow-up data.	3MS and Trails B Impairment defined as an 3MS score <80 or decline ≥5; or increase in Trails B time ≥1 SD above mean change.	Odds of incident impairment in relation to CKD was observed but was attenuated and not significant with adjustment for age.
3,154 INVADE study participants (>54 years) (396 with cognitive impairment at baseline and 194 with incident cognitive impairment at follow-up.	Blessed Information Memory Concentration Scale (6CIT). A score >7 defined as impairment.	eGFR <45 associated with cognitive impairment with adjustment for all covariates. With exclusion of CKD at baseline, incident CKD (eGFR <60) was associated with incident cognitive impairment (covariates not reported).

Table 4. Continued

Authors, outcome and time to follow-up	Predictor(s)	Controls: adjustments or exclusions
Seliger et al. [27] (2004) *Incident dementia* (AD and VaD); follow-up median 6 years.	Primary: 1/sCR. Secondary: renal insufficiency: sCR ≥1.3 mg/dl for women and 1.5 mg/dl for men.	Basic: adjustment for age, sex, race and body weight. Education, coronary heart disease, diabetes, hypertension, smoking status, and ApoE genotype; Exclusions: prevalent dementia at baseline.
Helmer et al. [23] (2011) *Incident dementia* (AD, vascular) and change in level of performance on the MMSE; follow-up median 6.8 years.	eGFR (CKD-EPI) at baseline and change in eGFR over time, proteinuria.	Basic: adjustment for study center, age, sex, education, APOE genotype. Additional: hypertension, CVD, stroke, high lipid levels, diabetes, smoking, BMI, baseline eGFR. Exclusions: prevalent dementia at baseline.
Sasaki et al. [26] (2011) *Incident dementia*	CKD present/absent based on eGFR and albuminuria.	Age, sex, education, hypertension, diabetes, dyslipidemia, ischemic heart disease, anemia.

[1] Negative results are not summarized (see variables column).

line to follow-up. However, a decline in renal function over time (indicated by eGFR or sCR) was related to a decline in global cognitive performance, verbal memory and abstract reasoning. Negative findings relative to decline in cognitive performance relative to baseline levels of renal function are not readily explained by study length or number of cognitive measures. Relative to other studies, Davey et al. [4] featured the largest number of cognitive outcomes and a fairly long follow-up of 4–5 years. But the sample was relatively well educated and change in renal function may be more sensitive in terms of cognitive change than baseline levels. Following 2,406 participants over 4 years, Helmer et al. [23] also found that change in renal function over 4 years but not baseline renal function was related to longitudinal decline (incident dementia).

None of the longitudinal studies used an everyday measure of cognitive performance or employed numeracy as a predictor or covariate and only 5 of the 16 studies summarized in tables 4 and 5 adjusted for clinical depression or depressed mood.

Obviously, there is a need for more studies with comprehensive test batteries, longer longitudinal follow-up periods and stratification by education level and/or numeracy skill, and with explicit exclusion of renal dialysis patients. Yet considering these studies collectively, it is clear that depending on severity of renal disease and the general health of the study population, various indices of

Sample	Cognitive tests or diagnostic category	Major statistically significant findings[1]
3,349 participants of the Cardiovascular Health Cognition Study (age> 64 years). Incident dementia = 477 cases. Stratification by health status at baseline: poor, good and excellent.	Diagnosis of dementia based on multiple test scores and clinical review. Type of dementia assessed with MRI.	Associations between elevated creatinine and incident dementia, but only for non- dementia participants in good to excellent health at baseline; higher sCR associated with increased risk of VaD, but not 'pure' AD-type dementia.
7,839 participants of the 3C Study (baseline eGFR); 2,382 multiple eGFR 1,040 proteinuria (age >65 years).	Diagnosis of dementia; based on NP examination and review by neurologist (DSM-IV criteria). Etiology based on NINCDS-ADRDA and NINDS-AIREN criteria.	No increased risk of cognitive decline or incident dementia in relation to eGFR at baseline. However, eGFR decline was associated with decline in global cognition (MMSE) and eGFR decline >4/year and proteinuria were related to increased risk for incident vascular dementia (with adjustment for extended covariate set).
256 community-dwelling participants from the Osaki-Tajiri Project (Northern Japan) (≥65 years).	Dementia: NINCDS-ADRDA and NINDS-AIREN criteria.	Association between CKD and conversion to dementia from a normal or questionable state at baseline with adjustment for all covariates.

CKD prevalence are related to decline in cognitive performance over time and dementia in samples over 65 years of age. What is not known from current studies is the prevalence, incidence or rate of cognitive decline prior to dementia.

It is encouraging to find that in the study of relatively well-educated nondemented community-based subjects, dialysis excluded, decline in performance levels over 4–5 years was modest and not such that they would interfere with understanding and adherence necessary to the treatment of renal disease [4].

Mechanisms Relating Kidney Disease to Cognition

Table 6 lists variables that may mediate between renal disease and cognitive function. One may hypothesize, among other models, direct paths in which CKD affects brain function and morphology and hence cognition. An alternative, and not mutually exclusive, possibility is that risk factors shared by brain and kidney lead to cognitive deficit, decline and impairment [30]. This parallel risk factor model is appealing because 'both kidney and brain are low resistance end organs and are exposed and re-exposed to high-volume blood flow though the cardiac cycle' [30, p. 5]. Thus the brain and kidney very likely share

Table 5. Summary check sheet for essential methods and findings with eGFR serum creatinine, albuminuria as outcome variables with studies ordered as in table 4

First author	eGFR	Creatinine	Albuminuria	MMSE/3MS (Global)	Composite of tests (Global)	Number of tests used as outcomes	Dementia	Decline on *any* test or incident dementia	
								relative to baseline renal function	relative to change in renal function
Buchman	✓			✓	✓	19		✓ eGFR	
Jassal	✓		✓	✓		2		✓ albuminuria male	
Wang	✓		✓	✓				✓ eGFR	
Davey	✓	✓			✓	19			✓ eGFR/sCR
Kurella	✓	✓		✓				✓	
Slinin	✓			✓		1			
Etgen[1]	✓					1		✓ eGFR	
Seliger[2, 3]		✓					✓	✓ eGFR/sCR	
Helmer	✓						✓		✓
Sasaki	✓						✓	✓	

[1] Based on Cockroft-Gault formula, standardized for body surface area.
[2] Renal insufficiency, defined differently for men (1.5 mg/dl) and women (1.3 mg/dl), was related incident dementia.
[3] Only for dementia-free persons in good or excellent health at baseline.

Table 6. Some candidate mechanisms mediating between kidney disease and cognitive functioning on order of discussion in text[1]

CVD risk factors	Hypertension, chronic hypotension, diabetes mellitus, hyperlipidemia, cardiovascular disease, including myocardial infarction, arterial fibrillation, cigarette smoking, elevated homocysteine, hemostatic abnormalities, hypercoagulation, oxidative stress, inflammation, acute stroke
Biologic intrinsic	Vascular changes in brain; anemia, white matter lesions, anemia, cortical atrophy, hyperparathyroidism, microalbuminuria, subclinical atherosclerosis
Psychosocial/treatment	Clinical depression and depressed mood and other psychosocial variables, polypharmacy, malnutrition
Dialysis-related	Hypotensive episodes, chronic microembolism, subclinical increases in brain edema, acute stroke, silent and asymptomatic stroke, hemodynamic changes and fluid shifts, microalbuminuria, recurrent cerebral ischemia, acute dynamic cardiovascular changes, lacunar infarcts, microbleeds

[1]See reviews of the literature including references 3–5.

common risk factors for cognitive deficit and impairment. It is clear that the issue of mediating variables becomes complex once treatment is initiated for ESRD. Thus we refer the reader to a comprehensive model by Murray and Knopman [5] and in table 6 summarize the many candidate mechanisms. In pretreatment forms of renal disease it makes some sense that the search for mechanisms should begin with the strongest risk factors for kidney disease, i.e. hypertension and diabetes. However, few if any mediation studies have been undertaken.

Methodological Issues

Controls

Controls for age, education, sex and, where relevant, race and ethnic composition are imperative, and controls for prevalent CVD risk factors, including depressed mood or clinical depression, and CVD events (e.g. acute stroke) are very important. But inspection of table 6 indicates that many other potential confounders exist even where the focus is pre-ESRD kidney disease. Polypharmacy is highly prevalent in the elderly. Moreover, many social psychological factors that are correlated with renal disease are especially important when patient groups or nonpatients are employed as control groups.

Cognitive Measurement

The finding that renal disease is related to multiple cognitive abilities, with few exceptions (e.g. over-learned crystallized intelligence), may be related to the fact that renal disease has a diffuse effect on brain function. However, it is important to recognize that the clinical cognitive tests traditionally employed in research on disease are impure, i.e., they measure a mixture of intended and untended cognitive constructs. Clinical cognitive tests are highly correlated with each other and with tests of general intellectual functioning [9]. There are two solutions: (1) factor analyses that identify theoretically-relevant cognitive domains [e.g. 19], and (2) utilization of more precise information processing tasks [9]. The latter method increases measurement purity but also increases performance difficulty for poorly educated study participants, makes significant demands on study time, and is less clinically interpretable.

Clinical Implications

In general, predialysis and pretransplant levels of cognitive deficit are relatively modest in well cared for and relatively highly educated, dementia- and stroke-free community samples [e.g. 19, 22]. This is good news and suggests that intervention might possibly be effective in preventing or delaying more serious ESRD and ESRD treatment-related cognitive deficit and impairment [5]. This conclusion is tentative pending more studies and clinical trials.

Conclusion

Prior to ESRD and treatment, kidney disease can result in global and multiple, specific-cognitive deficits, often mild, but sometimes associated with dementia. Treatment methods are improving but the physiological consequences of treatment can lead to more severe deficit. Biological factors intrinsic to renal disease, psychosocial factors, and polypharmacy are candidate intervening mechanisms, but formal studies identifying mediators between mild and modest levels of kidney disease and cognition have not been done.

We are starting down the path of a complex and challenging area of research and have a long way to go. We are in a descriptive phase of research, albeit we need more studies with comprehensive batteries of cognitive tests and tests of everyday cognitive function. To our knowledge, there have been no randomized-to-treatment clinical trials addressing improvement in cognitive performance with treatment for CVD risk factors. The clinical trial literature on hypertension provides a good model for this important next step.

Acknowledgements

This review was supported, in part, by grants R01HL67358 and R01HL081290 from the National Heart Lung and Blood Institute, National Institutes of Health (USA).

References

1 Alzheimer's Association: 2012 Alzheimer's disease facts and figures. Alzheimers Dement 2012;8:131–168.
2 Koushik NS, McArthur SF, Baird AD: Adult chronic kidney disease: neurocognition in chronic renal failure. Neuropsychol Rev 2010;20:33–51.
3 Etgen T, Chonchol M, Förstl H, Sander D: Chronic kidney disease and cognitive impairment: a systematic review and meta-analysis. Am J Nephrol 2012;35:474–482.
4 Davey A, Elias MF, Robbins MA, Seliger SL, Dore GA: Decline in renal functioning is associated with longitudinal decline in global cognitive functioning, abstract reasoning and verbal memory. Nephrol Dial Transplant 2012: Advance online publication. doi: 10.1093/ndt/gfs470.
5 Murray AM, Knopman DS: Cognitive impairment in CKD: no longer an occult burden. Am J Kidney Dis 2010;56:615–618.
6 Griva K, Stygall J, Hankins M, Davenport A, Harrison M, Newman SP: Cognitive impairment and 7-year mortality in dialysis patients. Am J Kidney Dis 2010;56:693–703.
7 National Kidney Foundation: Frequently asked questions about GFR estimates. NY, NY www.kidney.org.
8 Elias MF, Goodell AL, Dore GA: Hypertension and cognitive functioning: a perspective in historical context. Hypertension 2012;60: 260–268.
9 Rabbit P (ed): Methodology of Frontal and Executive Function. Hove, East Essex, UK: Psychology Press, 1998.
10 Radic J, Ljutic D, Radic M, Kovacid V, Sain M, Cukovic KD: The possible impact of dialysis modality on cognitive function in chronic dialysis patients. Neth J Med 2010;63: 153–157.

11 Abdel-Kader K, Dew MA, Bhatnagar M, Argyropoulos C, Karpov I, Switzer G, Unruh ML: Numeracy skills in CKD: correlates and outcomes. Clin J Am Soc Nephrol 2010;5:1566–1573.
12 Grubbs V, Gregorich SE, Perez-Stable EJ, Hsu CY: Health literacy and access to kidney transplantation. Clin J Am Soc Nephrol 2009;4:195–200.
13 Gelb SR, Shapiro RJ, Thornton WJ: Predicting medication adherence and employment status following kidney transplant: the relative utility of traditional and everyday cognitive approaches. Neuropsychology 2010;24:514–526.
14 Thornton WL, Shapiro RJ, Deria S, Gelb S, Hill A: Differential impact of age on verbal memory and executive functioning in chronic kidney disease. J Int Neuropsychol Soc 2007;13:344–353.
15 Hailpern SM, Melamed ML, Cohen HW, Hostetter TH: Moderate chronic kidney disease and cognitive function in adults 20 to 59 years of age: Third National Health and Nutrition Examination Survey (NHANES III). J Am Soc Nephrol 2007;18:2205–2213.
16 Kurella M, Yaffe K, Shlipak MG, Wenger NK, Chertow GM: Chronic kidney disease and cognitive impairment in menopausal women. Am J Kidney Dis 2005;45:66–76.
17 Jassal SV, Roscoe J, LeBlanc D, Devins GM, Rourke S: Differential impairment of psychomotor efficiency and processing speed in patients with chronic kidney disease. Int Urol Nephrol 2008;40:849–854.
18 Kurella Tamura M, Wadley V, Yaffe K, McKlure LA, Howard G, Go R, Warnock DG, McClellan W: Kidney function and cognitive impairment in US adults: the Reasons for Geographic and Racial Differences in Stroke (REGARDS) Study. Am J Kidney Dis 2008;52:227–234.
19 Elias MF, Elias PK, Seliger SL, Narsipur SS, Dore GA, Robbins MA: Chronic kidney disease, creatinine and cognitive functioning. Nephrol Dial Transplant 2009;24:2446–2452.
20 Etgen T, Sander D, Chonchol M, Briesenick C, Poppert H, Förstl H, Bickel H: Chronic kidney disease is associated with incident cognitive impairment in the elderly: the INVADE study. Nephrol Dial Transplant 2009;24:3144–3150.
21 Elias MF, Beiser A, Wolf PA, Au R, White RF, D'Agostino RB: The preclinical phase of Alzheimer disease: a 22-year prospective study of the Framingham Cohort. Arch Neurol 2000;57:808–813.
22 Buchman AS, Tanne D, Boyle PA, Shah RC, Leurgans SE, Bennett DA: Kidney function is associated with the rate of cognitive decline in the elderly. Neurology 2009;73:920–927.
23 Helmer C, Stengel B, Metzger M, Froissart M, Massy ZA, Tzourio C, Berr C, Dartigues JF: Chronic kidney disease, cognitive decline, and incident dementia: the 3C Study. Neurology 2011;77:2043–2051.
24 Jassal S, Kritz-Silverstein D, Barrett-Connor E: A prospective study of albuminuria and cognitive function in older adults: the Rancho Bernardo study. Am J Epidomiol 2010;171:277–286.
25 Kurella M, Chertow GM, Fried LF, Cummings SR, Harris T, Simonsick E, Satterfield S, Ayonayon H, Yaffe K: Chronic kidney disease and cognitive impairment in the elderly: the health, aging, and body composition study. J Am Soc Nephrol 2005;16:2127–2133.
26 Sasaki Y, Marioni R, Kasai M, Ishii H, Yamaguchi S, Meguro K: Chronic kidney disease: a risk factor for dementia onset: a population-based study. The Osaki-Tajiri Project. J Am Geriatr Soc 2011;59:1175–1181.
27 Seliger SL, Siscovick DS, Stehman-Breen CO, Gillen DL, Fitzpatrick A, Bleyer A, Kuller LH: Moderate renal impairment and risk of dementia among older adults: the Cardiovascular Health Cognition Study. J Am Soc Nephrol 2004;15:1904–1911.
28 Wang F, Zhang L, Liu L, Wang H: Level of kidney function correlates with cognitive decline. Am J Nephrol 2010;32:117–121.
29 Slinin Y, Paudel ML, Ishani A, Taylor BC, Yaffe K, Murray AM, Fink HA, Orwoll ES, Cummings SR, Conneer EB, Jassel S, Ensrud KE: Kidney function and cognitive performance and decline in older men. J Am Geriatr Soc 2008;56:2082–2088.
30 Seliger ST, Longsstreth WT Jr: Lessons about brain vascular diseases from another pulsating organ, the kidney. Stroke 2008;39:5–6.

Merrill F. Elias
Department of Psychology, The University of Maine
5742 Little Hall
Orono, ME 04469 (USA)
E-Mail MFElias@maine.edu

Toyoda K (ed): Brain, Stroke and Kidney.
Contrib Nephrol. Basel, Karger, 2013, vol 179, pp 58–66 (DOI: 10.1159/000346724)

Risk of Stroke in Kidney Disease

Toshiharu Ninomiya

Department of Medicine and Clinical Science, Graduate School of Medical Sciences,
Kyushu University, Fukuoka, Japan

Abstract

Stroke is a leading cause of mortality and morbidity worldwide. Traditional cardiovascular risk factors – hypertension, diabetes and dyslipidemia – are related to the incidence of stroke. Chronic kidney disease has also been recognized to be a major public health problem as a cardiovascular risk factor. Growing evidence has suggested that chronic kidney disease is associated with an increased risk of cardiovascular disease including stroke in general populations. Those with chronic kidney disease have a greater prevalence of traditional cardiovascular risk factors. Several meta-analyses assessing the association between chronic kidney disease and stroke have found that the magnitude of the risk estimates adjusted for known traditional cardiovascular risk factors were reduced as compared with the age-adjusted risk estimates. While these findings on the surface seem to downplay the effect of chronic kidney disease on stroke, they may actually suggest that an accumulation of traditional cardiovascular risk factors in those with chronic kidney disease increases the risk of stroke, and that applying appropriate treatments to those with chronic kidney disease is important for reducing the risk of stroke. Additionally, other large-scale meta-analyses demonstrated that chronic kidney disease was a significant risk factor for stroke independent of known cardiovascular risk factors. Chronic kidney disease may also be associated with an increase in nontraditional risk factors such as hyperhomocysteinemia, inflammation, asymmetric dimethylarginine, oxidative stress, and anemia, and thrombogenic factors such as left ventricular hypertrophy, endothelial dysfunction, and arterial stiffness. Herein, we review the results of meta-analyses of published cohort studies for a better understanding of the precise nature of the relationship between chronic kidney disease and stroke, important to both the clinical and public health fields. Further studies are warranted to determine whether interventions to prevent the progression of kidney impairment are effective at reducing the risk of stroke.

Stroke is a leading cause of mortality and morbidity worldwide [1]. It has been well recognized that the traditional cardiovascular risk factors, namely hypertension, diabetes and dyslipidemia, contribute to the etiology of stroke [2–4].

Therefore, the optimal management of these risk factors has been known to be effective for preventing the development of stroke.

It is now understood that chronic kidney disease, most commonly defined by a reduction in the estimated glomerular filtration rate (eGFR) or the presence of proteinuria, presents a major public health problem, especially as a cardiovascular risk factor. Growing evidence from numerous epidemiological studies suggests that reduced eGFR and elevated proteinuria are associated with an increased risk of all-cause and cardiovascular mortality in general populations [5]. As those with chronic kidney disease have a greater prevalence of traditional cardiovascular risk factors, it may be important that appropriate treatments, such as blood pressure- and glucose-lowering therapy and use of statins can be applied to those with chronic kidney disease for reducing the risk of cardiovascular disease including stroke.

Herein, we review the results of meta-analyses of published cohort studies for a better understanding of the precise nature of the relationship between chronic kidney disease and stroke, to provide insights to both clinical and public health fields.

Relationship between Reduced eGFR and Stroke

Kidney disease and stroke share traditional cardiovascular risk factors, such as aging, diabetes, hypertension and hyperlipidemia [6]. Therefore, kidney dysfunction may simply be a marker for the duration or severity of traditional cardiovascular risk factors. There is conflicting evidence as to whether reduced eGFR is a risk factor for stroke independent of traditional cardiovascular risk factors [7, 8].

In a pooled analysis using 22,634 subjects from community-based longitudinal studies including the ARIC Study, Cardiovascular Health Study, Framingham Heart Study, and Framingham Offspring Study, subjects with eGFR below 60 ml/min/1.73 m^2 had a higher incidence of stroke, at 10.3 events per 1,000 person-years, than those with eGFR above 60 ml/min/1.73 m^2 (3.4 events per 1,000 person-years). However, reduced eGFR was not a significant risk factor for stroke after adjusting for cardiovascular risk factors (HR 1.17, 95% CI 0.95–1.44) [9]. On the other hand, a subgroup analysis of this study among the 4,278 subjects with preexisting cardiovascular disease identified that subjects with eGFR of <60 ml/min/1.73 m^2 were at 1.30-fold (95% CI 1.04–1.63) increased risk for stroke after adjusting for traditional cardiovascular risk factors. Likewise, in a pooled analysis using 30,657 individual participant data from 10 community-based cohort studies in Japan, the age- and sex-adjusted hazard ratios (HRs) of the development of stroke increased gradually with lower eGFR levels, being 1.40 (95% CI 1.10–1.79) and 2.06 (95% CI 1.51–2.81) in subjects with eGFRs of 60–89 and <60 ml/min/1.73 m^2, respectively [10]. Again, the effect of reduced eGFR on the risk of stroke was not significant (HR 1.24 [95% CI 0.95–1.61] and HR 1.41 [95% CI 0.99–2.00] for eGFRs of 60–89, and <60 ml/min/1.73 m^2) after adjusting for the traditional risk factors including blood pressure, diabetes, serum total cholesterol, body mass index, and smoking habits. These findings suggest that the increased risk of stroke among subjects with reduced eGFR was mainly attributable to an accumulation of traditional cardiovascular risk factors, although the possible involvement of 'novel' risk factors could not be denied.

Stroke is common in dialysis patients. The risk of stroke in these patients has been found to be 4–10 times higher than that in the general population [11]. Of interest is the finding of one study that stroke events early after starting dialysis therapy were likely to develop in patients with kidney failure caused by either nephrosclerosis or diabetes mellitus, whereas most patients with chronic glomerulonephritis experienced stroke events more than 36 months after starting dialysis therapy [12]. Supportive findings from a chronic kidney disease Japan cohort study of 2,977 patients with eGFR of 10–59 ml/min/1.73 m^2 showed that patients with diabetic nephropathy or nonchronic glomerulonephritic kidney disease had a greater brachial-ankle pulse wave velocity, which is a marker of atherosclerotic disease, than those with chronic glomerulonephritis [13]. This finding supports the data that perhaps kidney impairment in combination with other cardiovascular risk factors accelerates atherosclerosis and raises the risk of the development of stroke in the predialysis stages.

On the other hand, several studies have indicated that an elevated risk for stroke in subjects with lower eGFR independent of other traditional cardiovascular risk factors [14–17]. A hospital-based study of 6,685 Israeli patients with chronic coronary heart found that those with eGFR below 60 ml/min/1.73 m^2 had a 1.53-fold increased risk (95% CI 1.16–2.01) for incident stroke or TIA; the corresponding adjusted hazard ratio (HR) associated with a decrement of 1 SD in eGFR was 1.19 (95% CI 1.05–1.33) [16]. A community-based cohort study conducted in 5,494 Japanese individuals aged 30–79 years demonstrated that the multivariate-adjusted HRs for stroke were 1.94 (95% CI 1.26–2.98) in those with eGFR 50–59 ml/min/1.73 m^2 and 2.19 (95% CI 1.18–4.06) in those with eGFR of <50 ml/min/1.73 m^2, as compared to those with eGFR of ≥90 ml/min/1.73 m^2 [17]. The same was true for ischemic stroke. The Atherosclerosis Risk in Communities (ARIC) study assessed the joint effect of kidney disease and anemia on the risk for incident stroke [18]. This study of a general population in USA found that a low kidney function defined as creatinine clearance of <60 ml/min was associated with a 1.81-fold (95% CI 1.26–2.02) increased risk for stroke after adjusting for cardiovascular risk factors. Additionally, a subgroup analysis of patients with anemia found that the magnitude of the effect of low kidney function was greater in the presence of anemia (HR 5.43, 95% CI 2.04–14.41), with only a modest increased risk in the presence of a normal hemoglobin level (HR 1.41, 95% CI 0.93–2.14): the interaction between kidney disease and anemia on the risk of stroke was statistically significant ($p < 0.01$).

The recent meta-analysis of 21 articles derived from 33 prospective studies among 284,672 people experiencing 7,863 stroke events, in which multivariate-adjusted relative risks (RRs) were pooled, suggested that the risk of incident stroke increased by 43% (95% CI 31–57%) in subjects with an eGFR of <60 ml/min/1.73 m^2, but not in those with an eGFR of 60–90 ml/min/1.73 m^2 (RR 1.07, 95% CI 0.98–1.17) (fig. 1) [19]. There was a significant heterogeneity in the risk estimates of an eGFR of <60 ml/min/1.73 m^2 across the studies included ($p < 0.001$). Reduced eGFR was a risk factor for both ischemic and hemorrhagic stroke, without evidence of heterogeneity in the association between stroke subtypes (p for heterogeneity = 0.10). A total of 11 studies from studies included in this meta-analysis reported both age- and sex-adjusted estimates of the strength of the association between eGFR <60 ml/min/1.73 m^2 and the risk estimates adjusted for other known cardiovascular risk factors. As a consequence, the age- and sex-adjusted summary estimates was 1.64 (95% CI 1.45–1.85), which after further adjustment for other cardiovascular risk factors was reduced to 1.45 (95% 1.26–1.68) with the evidence of significant heterogeneity between the risk estimates (p for heterogeneity = 0.01). Interestingly, this meta-analysis found that the impact of an eGFR of <60 ml/min/1.73 m^2 was significantly greater in Asian populations (RR 1.96, 95% CI 1.73–2.23) than in non-Asian populations (RR 1.26, 95% CI 1.16–1.35; p for heterogeneity <0.001). Certainly, hypertension is a major risk factor for stroke among Asian populations, and the risk of stroke associated with hypertension is significantly greater in Asian people than in Caucasians [20, 21].

Relationship between Proteinuria and Stroke

Several prospective studies have suggested that the presence of protein in the urine ('albuminuria' or 'proteinuria') is directly associated with cardiovascular events including stroke [22–25]. However, there was evidence of a relatively small amount of heterogeneity in the magnitude of the association between proteinuria and the risk of stroke across the studies. A meta-analysis of 10 prospective cohort studies involving 140,231 participants and 3,266 stroke events suggested that subjects with proteinuria had a 71% (95% CI 39–110%) greater risk of stroke compared with those without proteinuria (fig. 2). The risk for stroke

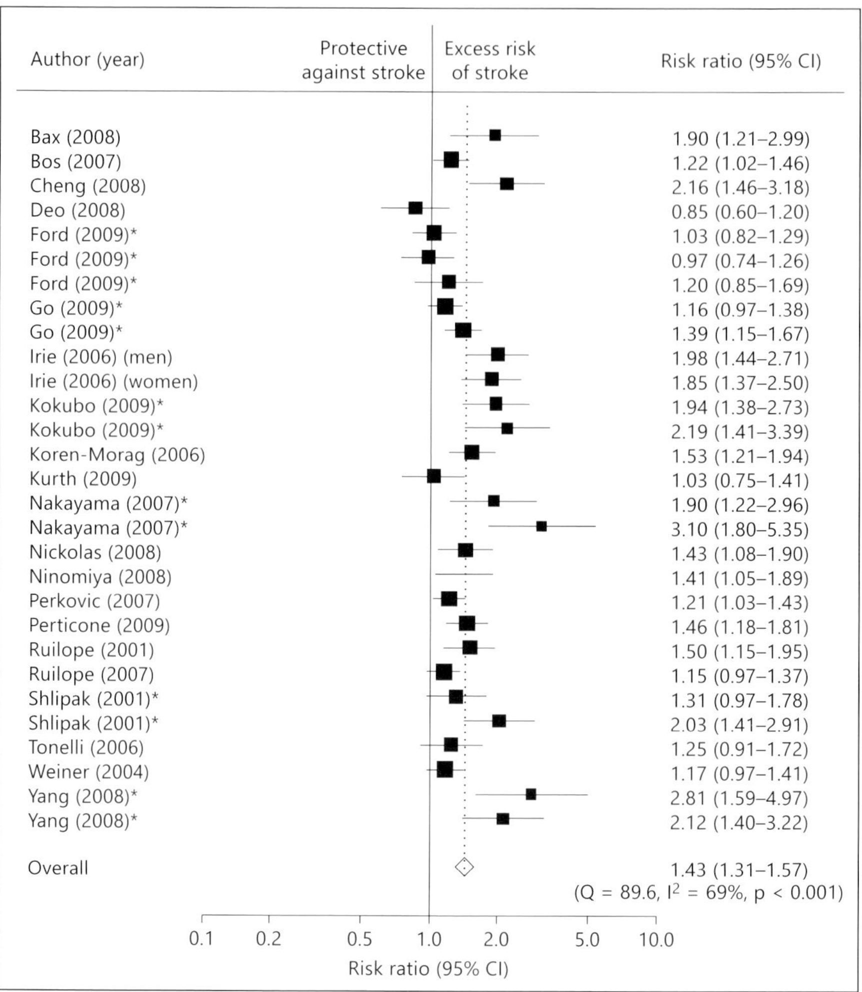

Fig. 1. Overall risk ratio for association of estimated glomerular filtration rate of <60 ml/min/1.73 m^2 with the risk of stroke in prospective cohort studies. From Lee et al. [19]. * Subgroups of estimates with eGFR <60 ml/min/1.73 m^2.

remained significant after adjustment for other vascular risk factors [26]. There was evidence of significant quantitative heterogeneity in the magnitude of the association across studies (p for heterogeneity = 0.008), which was partially explained by differences in the method for measuring proteinuria (dipstick or laboratory measuring method). Additionally, comparison of the summary estimates from the studies that reported both age- and multivariate-adjusted estimates showed that the relationship between proteinuria and stroke was attenuated by 30% after adjusting for known cardiovascular risk factors (RR 2.81 [95% CI 1.78–4.42] vs. RR 1.94 [95% CI 1.37–2.75]).

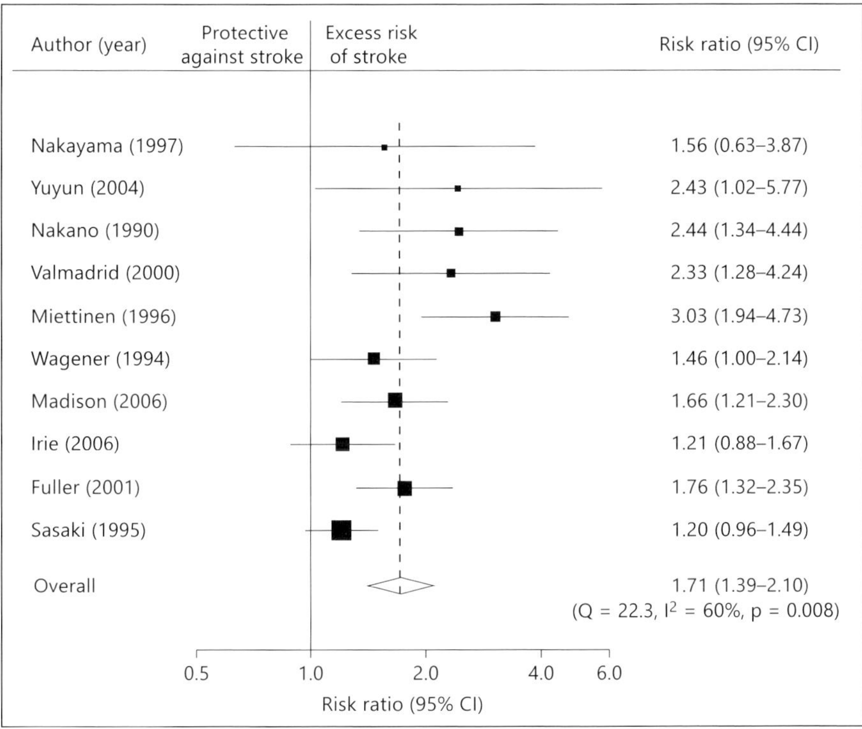

Fig. 2. Overall risk ratio for association of proteinuria with the risk of stroke in prospective cohort studies. From Ninomiya et al. [26].

Data in support of a role for proteinuria in stroke are derived from post hoc analyses of large-scale clinical trials which suggest that reducing the level of albuminuria is associated with a concurrent reduction in cardiovascular risk. In the Reduction in Endpoints in Non-insulin-dependent diabetes mellitus with the Angiotensin II Antagonist Losartan (RENAAL) study, involving 1,500 patients with type II diabetes mellitus and nephropathy, a 50% reduction in albuminuria was associated with a significant 18% reduction in the risk of cardiovascular disease [27]. Similarly, in the Losartan Intervention for Endpoint Reduction in Hypertension (LIFE) Study, among 8,200 patients with hypertension and left ventricular hypertrophy, participants who achieved a lower level of albuminuria using losartan or atenolol-based regimens had a significantly lower risk of subsequent fatal or nonfatal stroke than those with persistent albuminuria [28]. Although these associations do not necessarily imply causality and are potentially confounded by parallel changes in blood pressure, they suggest that reductions in urinary protein excretion may result in a reduction in the risk of subsequent stroke events.

These findings support the hypothesis that proteinuria is an independent risk factor for stroke. Routine measurement of urinary protein may therefore improve current tools for the assessment and modification of stroke risk. Further studies are warranted to determine whether interventions to reduce proteinuria are effective at reducing rates of stroke.

Possible Mechanisms Underlying the Relationship between CKD and Stroke

There are several possible explanations for the association of reduced GFR with stroke [29]. As mentioned above, reduced GFR is associated with a high prevalence of traditional cardiovascular risk factors, such as aging, hypertension, diabetes, smoking habits, and dyslipidemia. Several meta-analyses assessing the association between CKD and stroke found that the magnitude of the risk estimates were reduced after adjusting for known traditional cardiovascular risk factors as compared with age-adjusted risk estimates. These findings suggest that an accumulation of traditional cardiovascular risk factors in subjects with CKD increases the risk of stroke. Additionally, large-scale meta-analyses demonstrated that CKD was a significant risk factor for stroke, independent of known cardiovascular risk factors [19, 26]. CKD may also be associated with an increase in other nontraditional risk factors such as hyperhomocysteinemia, inflammation, asymmetric dimethylarginine, oxidative stress, anemia, thrombogenic factors, left ventricular hypertrophy, endothelial dysfunction, and arterial stiffness [30]. On the other hand, CKD may be a marker for both the duration and severity of other causes of stroke, such as hypertension and diabetes. Last, the results from several previous studies may imply either that CKD itself is a causal factor in the pathogenesis of stroke, or that CKD is simply a marker of cerebral small vessel pathology. The kidney and brain share unique susceptibilities to vascular injury, so that some vascular risk factors like hypertension, diabetes, and heart disease may cause similar vascular injuries in both organs.

Conclusions

The data from epidemiological studies support the hypothesis that both reduced eGFR and increased urinary proteinuria are independent risk factors for stroke. Routine measurement of both eGFR and urinary protein may therefore improve current tools for the assessment and modification of stroke risk. Further studies are warranted to determine whether interventions to prevent the progression of kidney impairment are effective at reducing the risk of stroke.

References

1 Prevention WicwtUCfDCa: The Atlas of Heart Disease and Stroke. Global burden of stroke. http://www.who.int/cardiovascular_diseases/resources/atlas/en/index.html.

2 Executive Summary of the Third Report of the National Cholesterol Education Program (NCEP) Expert Panel on Detection, Evaluation, and Treatment of High Blood Cholesterol in Adults (Adult Treatment Panel III). JAMA 2001;285:2486–2497.

3 Asia Pacific Cohort Studies Collaboration: Joint effects of systolic blood pressure and serum cholesterol on cardiovascular disease in the Asia Pacific region. Circulation 2005; 112:3384–3390.

4 Woodward M, Zhang X, Barzi F, Pan W, Ueshima H, Rodgers A, et al: The effects of diabetes on the risks of major cardiovascular diseases and death in the Asia-Pacific region. Diabetes Care 2003;26:360–366.

5 Matsushita K, van der Velde M, Astor BC, Woodward M, Levey AS, de Jong PE, et al: Association of estimated glomerular filtration rate and albuminuria with all-cause and cardiovascular mortality in general population cohorts: a collaborative meta-analysis. Lancet 2010;375:2073–2081.

6 Goldstein LB, Adams R, Alberts MJ, Appel LJ, Brass LM, Bushnell CD, et al: Primary prevention of ischemic stroke: a guideline from the American Heart Association/American Stroke Association Stroke Council: cosponsored by the Atherosclerotic Peripheral Vascular Disease Interdisciplinary Working Group; Cardiovascular Nursing Council; Clinical Cardiology Council; Nutrition, Physical Activity, and Metabolism Council; and the Quality of Care and Outcomes Research Interdisciplinary Working Group: the American Academy of Neurology affirms the value of this guideline. Stroke 2006;37:1583–1633.

7 Culleton BF, Larson MG, Wilson PW, Evans JC, Parfrey PS, Levy D: Cardiovascular disease and mortality in a community-based cohort with mild renal insufficiency. Kidney Int 1999;56:2214–2219.

8 Garg AX, Clark WF, Haynes RB, House AA: Moderate renal insufficiency and the risk of cardiovascular mortality: results from the NHANES I. Kidney Int 2002;61:1486–1494.

9 Weiner DE, Tighiouart H, Amin MG, Stark PC, MacLeod B, Griffith JL, et al: Chronic kidney disease as a risk factor for cardiovascular disease and all-cause mortality: a pooled analysis of community-based studies. J Am Soc Nephrol 2004;15:1307–1315.

10 Ninomiya T, Kiyohara Y, Tokuda Y, Doi Y, Arima H, Harada A, et al: Impact of kidney disease and blood pressure on the development of cardiovascular disease: an overview from the Japan Arteriosclerosis Longitudinal Study. Circulation 2008;118:2694–2701.

11 Seliger SL, Gillen DL, Longstreth WT Jr, Kestenbaum B, Stehman-Breen CO: Elevated risk of stroke among patients with end-stage renal disease. Kidney Int 2003;64:603–609.

12 van der Sande FM, Hermans MM, Leunissen KM, Kooman JP. Noncardiac consequences of hypertension in hemodialysis patients. Semin Dial 2004;17:304–306.

13 Imai E, Matsuo S, Makino H, Watanabe T, Akizawa T, Nitta K, et al: Chronic Kidney Disease Japan Cohort study: baseline characteristics and factors associated with causative diseases and renal function. Clin Exp Nephrol 2010;14:558–570.

14 Henry RM, Kostense PJ, Bos G, Dekker JM, Nijpels G, Heine RJ, et al: Mild renal insufficiency is associated with increased cardiovascular mortality: The Hoorn Study. Kidney Int 2002;62:1402–1407.

15 Ninomiya T, Kiyohara Y, Kubo M, Tanizaki Y, Doi Y, Okubo K, et al: Chronic kidney disease and cardiovascular disease in a general Japanese population: the Hisayama Study. Kidney Int 2005;68:228–236.

16 Koren-Morag N, Goldbourt U, Tanne D: Renal dysfunction and risk of ischemic stroke or TIA in patients with cardiovascular disease. Neurology 2006;67:224–228.

17 Kokubo Y, Nakamura S, Okamura T, Yoshimasa Y, Makino H, Watanabe M, et al: Relationship between blood pressure category and incidence of stroke and myocardial infarction in an urban Japanese population with and without chronic kidney disease: the Suita Study. Stroke 2009;40:2674–2679.

18 Abramson JL, Jurkovitz CT, Vaccarino V, Weintraub WS, McClellan W: Chronic kidney disease, anemia, and incident stroke in a middle-aged, community-based population: the ARIC Study. Kidney Int 2003;64:610–615.

19 Lee M, Saver JL, Chang KH, Liao HW, Chang SC, Ovbiagele B: Low glomerular filtration rate and risk of stroke: meta-analysis. BMJ 2010;341:c4249.
20 Woodward M, Huxley H, Lam TH, Barzi F, Lawes CM, Ueshima H: A comparison of the associations between risk factors and cardiovascular disease in Asia and Australasia. Eur J Cardiovasc Prevent Rehab 2005; 12:484–491.
21 Zhang XF, Attia J, D'Este C, Ma XY: The relationship between higher blood pressure and ischaemic, haemorrhagic stroke among Chinese and Caucasians: meta-analysis. Eur J Cardiovasc Prevent Rehab 2006;13:429–437.
22 Valmadrid CT, Klein R, Moss SE, Klein BE: The risk of cardiovascular disease mortality associated with microalbuminuria and gross proteinuria in persons with older-onset diabetes mellitus. Arch Intern Med 2000;160: 1093–1100.
23 Miettinen H, Haffner SM, Lehto S, Ronnemaa T, Pyorala K, Laakso M: Proteinuria predicts stroke and other atherosclerotic vascular disease events in nondiabetic and non-insulin-dependent diabetic subjects. Stroke 1996;27:2033–2039.
24 Madison JR, Spies C, Schatz IJ, Masaki K, Chen R, Yano K, et al: Proteinuria and risk for stroke and coronary heart disease during 27 years of follow-up: the Honolulu Heart Program. Arch Intern Med 2006; 166:884–889.
25 Irie F, Iso H, Sairenchi T, Fukasawa N, Yamagishi K, Ikehara S, et al: The relationships of proteinuria, serum creatinine, glomerular filtration rate with cardiovascular disease mortality in Japanese general population. Kidney Int 2006;69:1264–1271.
26 Ninomiya T, Perkovic V, Verdon C, Barzi F, Cass A, Gallagher M, et al: Proteinuria and stroke: a meta-analysis of cohort studies. Am J Kidney Dis 2009;53:417–425.
27 de Zeeuw D, Remuzzi G, Parving HH, Keane WF, Zhang Z, Shahinfar S, et al: Albuminuria, a therapeutic target for cardiovascular protection in type 2 diabetic patients with nephropathy. Circulation 2004;110:921–927.
28 Ibsen H, Olsen MH, Wachtell K, Borch-Johnsen K, Lindholm LH, Mogensen CE, et al: Reduction in albuminuria translates to reduction in cardiovascular events in hypertensive patients: losartan intervention for endpoint reduction in hypertension study. Hypertension 2005;45:198–202.
29 Sarnak MJ, Levey AS, Schoolwerth AC, Coresh J, Culleton B, Hamm LL, et al: Kidney disease as a risk factor for development of cardiovascular disease: a statement from the American Heart Association Councils on Kidney in Cardiovascular Disease, High Blood Pressure Research, Clinical Cardiology, and Epidemiology and Prevention. Circulation 2003;108:2154–2169.
30 Sarnak MJ, Levey AS: Cardiovascular disease and chronic renal disease: a new paradigm. Am J Kidney Dis 2000;35(suppl 1):S117–S131.

Toshiharu Ninomiya, MD, PhD
Department of Medicine and Clinical Science
Graduate School of Medical Sciences, Kyushu University
3-1-1 Maidashi, Higashi-ku, Fukuoka City 812-8582 (Japan)
E-Mail nino@intmed2.med.kyushu-u.ac.jp

Toyoda K (ed): Brain, Stroke and Kidney.
Contrib Nephrol. Basel, Karger, 2013, vol 179, pp 67–80 (DOI: 10.1159/000346725)

Role of 24-Hour Blood Pressure Management in Preventing Kidney Disease and Stroke

Michiaki Nagai · Satoshi Hoshide · Kazuomi Kario

Division of Cardiovascular Medicine, Department of Medicine, Jichi Medical University School of Medicine, Tochigi, Japan

Abstract

Apart from the well-known role of hypertension in cerebrovascular disease, chronic kidney disease is emerging as an independent risk factor for stroke. Although the mechanism underlying the relationship between blood pressure variability, diurnal blood pressure variation disruption (e.g. nondipping) and kidney dysfunction is not fully understood, these factors are closely associated with each other. This review article summarizes the recent literature on these topics. Cerebral small vessel disease is considered to serve as a common pathophysiology in the relationship of hypertension and chronic kidney disease with cognitive impairment and stroke. Strict 24-hour blood pressure control is necessary to prevent the progression of kidney dysfunction, dementia and stroke.

Vascular disease of the brain is a major cause of death and disability [1]. Hypertension is the most potent risk factor for cardiovascular disease (CVD), including stroke, coronary artery disease, and chronic kidney disease (CKD). CKD has emerged as another independent risk factor for stroke and other cardiovascular events [2–4].

Ambulatory blood pressure monitoring (ABPM) was shown to provide a better predictive value for cardiovascular events than clinic blood pressure (BP) measurement [5]. In addition, ambulatory blood pressure (ABP) has been shown to have a closer correlation with target organ damage including kidney dysfunction and silent cerebral vascular disease.

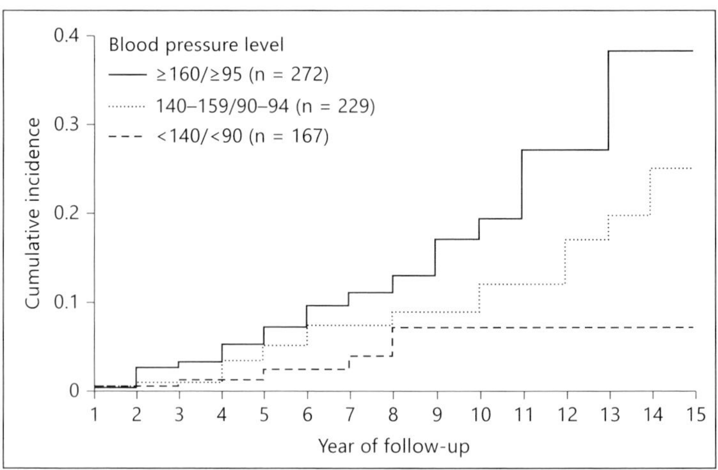

Fig. 1. Cumulative incidence of early kidney function decline among hypertensive men by level of BP. From Vupputuri et al. [11].

Magnetic resonance imaging (MRI) has revealed that white matter lesions are common in the elderly [6]. White matter hyperintensity (WMH) has been shown to be associated with stroke [7]. Hypertension is a well-known risk for WMH [8, 9]. Recently, CKD was also suggested as a risk factor of WMH [10].

From these perspectives, the relationships among hypertension, CKD and stroke have clinical relevance. The present review is aimed at thoroughly elucidating the research-derived associations between 24-hour BP, CKD and stroke. To set the stage, we summarize current insights into these relationships, and propose an updated explanation of the pathophysiology of the association of hypertension with CKD and stroke.

Hypertension, Chronic Kidney Disease and Stroke

Hypertensive patients have a greater decline in glomerular filtration rate (GFR) compared with normotensives (fig. 1) [11].

Ninomiya et al. [12] conducted follow-up on a total of 30,657 individuals 40–89 years of age. During an average 7.4-year follow-up, 727 individuals experienced CVD. The age- and sex-adjusted incidence of CVD increased significantly in subjects with GFR of 60–89 ml/min/1.73 m^2 (4.3 per 1,000 person-years, $p = 0.002$) and in those with a GFR <60 ml/min/1.73 m^2 (6.5, $p < 0.001$) compared with those with a GFR ≥90 ml/min/1.73 m^2. The multivariate-adjusted hazard ratios of CVD significantly increased in a log-linear manner with elevations in BP levels regardless of GFR levels, although a stronger association between BP and CVD was found in subjects with CKD.

Kokubo et al. [13] studied 5,494 Japanese individuals aged 30–79 years. During an average 11.7-year follow-up, 346 individuals experienced CVD. Compared with the optimal BP subjects without CKD, the normal BP, high-normal BP, and hypertensive subjects without CKD showed increased risks of CVD and stroke. The impact of each BP category on CVD (p for interaction: 0.04 in men, 0.49 in women) and stroke (0.03 in men, 0.90 in women) was more evident in men with CKD.

Overall, epidemiological studies in the Japanese population have suggested that CKD increases the association of BP and stroke.

Ambulatory Blood Pressure and Kidney

CKD is likely to exhibit a nondipping pattern of nocturnal BP falls [14], and this nondipping pattern might precede microalbuminuria [15]. It becomes evident that in patients with high-sodium sensitivity, the nocturnal dip in BP is diminished irrespective of the mechanisms causing sodium sensitivity [16].

Because glomerular filtration capability is one of the major factors determining sodium sensitivity, the nocturnal BP dip may be less pronounced as a function of GFR loss [17]. As GFR was reduced, the night-to-day ratio of BP, natriuresis, and proteinuria were all increased. Circadian BP rhythm is well known to be shifted to the nondipping pattern in CKD.

On the other hand, the nondipping pattern is often considered to be a risk for the progression of nephropathy [15]. Among the young with type 1 diabetes, nondippers more frequently develop albuminuria and latent nephropathy [15]. The rate in GFR decline was faster in nondippers than in dippers. As seen in the link between kidney disease and hypertension, renal dysfunction and nondipper status might be closely associated with each other.

Blood Pressure Variability, Stroke and Cognitive Impairment

BP levels are strong predictors of first and recurrent strokes [18, 19]. Average BP over a period of time is widely considered to be important as a cause of vascular disease [19]. On the other hand, in a large cohort of patients with a history of transient ischemic attacks (TIA; UK-TIA Aspirin Trials), and in a broad population of patients with hypertension in the Anglo-Scandinavian Cardiac Outcomes Trial Blood Pressure Lowering Arm (ASCOT-BPLA), Rothwell et al. [20]

reported that visit-to-visit systolic blood pressure (SBP) variability and maximum SBP were strong predictors of stroke, independent of average SBP.

Recently, we have shown that visit-to-visit BP variability was a significant indicator for carotid artery atherosclerosis and stiffness in the elderly at high risk of CVD [21]. Brickman et al. [22] reported that WMH volume was increased in the elderly with high BP and high visit-to-visit BP variability.

Although hypertension is a risk factor for vascular dementia [23, 24], trials of BP-lowering drugs have not shown a consistent reduction in the risk of dementia [25–27]. Most of the studies have been focused on absolute BP levels in relation with cognitive dysfunction or dementia. On the other hand, in the Kungsholmen Project, a greater decline in SBP occurring 3–6 years before diagnosis was associated with an increased risk of dementia in the elderly [28]. In the Honolulu Heart Program/Honolulu-Asia Aging Study, which had a 32-year follow-up period, the subjects who developed dementia had a greater SBP increase that was followed by a greater SBP decrease compared with those who did not [24].

In the ASCOT-BPLA ABPM study, daytime BP variability assessed by ABPM was correlated with clinic visit-to-visit BP variability [20]. That result might indicate that the strength of the association of visit-to-visit BP variability with cognitive function might be similar to that of daytime BP variability. In an earlier study, Sakakura et al. [29] showed that daytime SBP variability in the ABPM was negatively associated with the mini mental state examination (MMSE) score in the elderly.

In the HiroShima-Shobara-Soryo COhort (3SCO) study [30], we investigated the relationship between visit-to-visit BP variations and cognitive function among 201 elderly at high risk of CVD (79.9 ± 6.4 years old; females, 75%; antihypertensive medication use, 71%). Exaggerated long-term visit-to-visit BP fluctuations were significantly associated with lower MMSE scores (fig. 2), higher GDS scores, and cognitive impairment independently of average BP in the elderly at high- risk of CVD. Specifically, the CV SBP and delta SBP were significantly positively correlated with cognitive impairment in multiple regression models.

Ambulatory Blood Pressure and Silent Cerebral Ischemia

Silent Cerebral Infarcts

Silent cerebral infarction (SCI) is a strong surrogate marker of clinical stroke [31, 32]. Shimada et al. [33] have reported that non-dipping status was correlated with SCI in elderly hypertensives. In the JMS-ABPM Study, extreme dipping

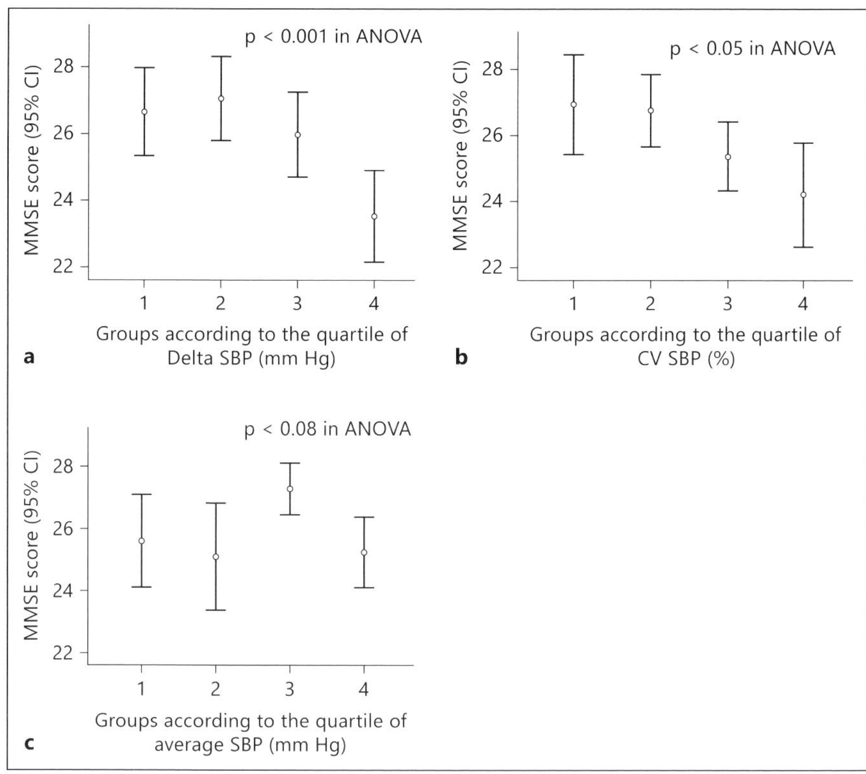

Fig. 2. Visit-to-visit BP variations and MMSE score. Mean MMSE score is presented according to the quartiles of Delta SBP (**a**), CV SBP (**b**), and average SBP (**c**). ANOVA was used to determine differences among 4 groups.From Nagai et al. [30].

and riser patterns were related with SCI as well as clinical stroke [31, 34]. Extreme dipping was suggested to be associated with cerebral hypoperfusion during sleep or an exaggerated morning BP rise, whereas riser status might pose a risk for intracranial hemorrhage. SCIs were more frequently detected in the morning surge group than in the nonsurge group [35].

White Matter Hyperintensity

Diminished nocturnal BP dip has been observed in patients with Binswanger disease [36]. Additionally, high ambulatory SBP level, exaggerated ABP variability, and prothrombotic status has been associated with progression of WMH [37, 38].

In the sibships of subjects in the Genetic Epidemiology Network Of Arteriopathy (GENOA) study, both SBP and diastolic BP (DBP) over 24-hour and

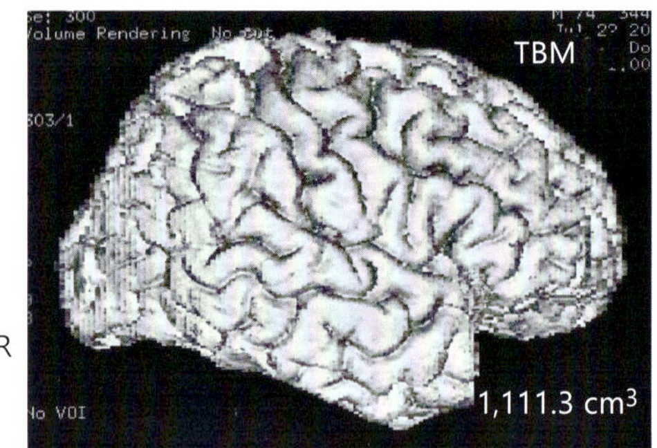

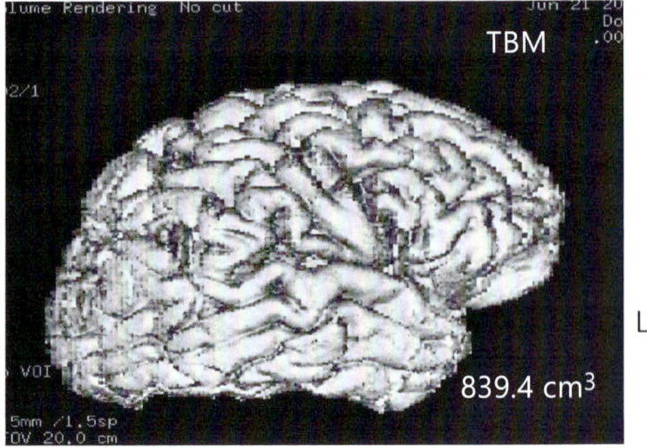

74-year-old male
24-hour SBP: 124 mm Hg
Awake SBP: 139 mm Hg
Sleep SBP: 118 mm Hg

Nocturnal SBP dipping: 15%
MMSE score: 29

73-year-old male
24-hour SBP: 144 mm Hg
Awake SBP: 138 mm Hg
Sleep SBP: 158 mm Hg

Nocturnal SBP dipping: –14%
MMSE score: 22

Fig. 3. Examples of 3D reconstructed images. On the left is an image of reconstructed TBM of a subject with normal nocturnal SBP fall. On the right is an image of reconstructed TBM of a subject with nocturnal SBP elevation. From Nagai et al. [45].

during the waking and sleeping periods were significantly positively associated with WMH volume in African-Caribbeans, while both nocturnal SBP and DBP dipping were significantly negatively associated with WMH volume among Caucasians [39]. Among the hypertensives, African-Caribbeans had significantly higher 24-hour SBP and DBP levels, greater parieto-occipital WMH volume, and poorer performance on executive function and verbal fluency than the Caucasians [40].

In a 2-year follow-up study, White et al. [41] revealed that an increase in 24-hour SBP from baseline was a predictor of increased WMH volume in the high risk elderly. In the 3C-Dijon Magnetic Imaging Study [42], subjects with antihypertensive treatment had a smaller increase in WMH volume at a 4-year follow-up than those without hypertensive treatment.

Brain Atrophy

Brain atrophy as assessed by MRI has been shown to be present in essential hypertensives [43]. In addition, 24-hour SBP has been shown to be an independent determinant for brain atrophy in the healthy elderly [44].

In the Jichi Medical School ABPM Study, Wave 2 Core, we performed ABPM and brain MRI in 55 unmedicated elderly hypertensives (fig. 3). Cognitive function was assessed with MMSE. Total brain matter (TBM) volume was significantly different among the three tertiles of MMSE score. In particular, the low-MMSE-score group had significantly lower TBM volume than the high-MMSE-score group. In multiple linear regression analysis adjusted for age, sex and BMI, sleep SBP was more significantly negatively associated with TBM volume than was either 24-hour or awake SBP [45]. Similarly, Hajjar et al. [46] have reported that nondipping status was associated with brain atrophy.

Although several contradictory findings have been observed in regard to the pathophysiology of the relationship between ABP variation disruption and cognitive impairment [47, 48], the results suggest that WML or brain atrophy can serve as determinants for brain damage progression.

Kidney and White Matter Hyperintensity

WMH has been shown to be more prevalent in patients with end-stage renal disease [49]. In addition, CKD has also been linked to proinflammatory and procoagulant states [50, 51] that may contribute to WMH development [52, 53].

In the Northern Manhattan Study (NOMAS), moderate-to-severe CKD was associated with increased WML volume, proving the importance of CKD as a possible marker of cerebral microangiopathy [10]. In the Genetics of Microangiopathic Brain Injury (GMBI) Study, an elevated urine albumin/creatinine ratio was independently associated with both brain atrophy and increased WMH volume [54]. In the Aging, and Memory in Elders (NAME) study, albuminuria was associated with an increased WMH volume in the elderly [55].

Like microalbuminuria, decreased GFR is often attributable to renal small vessel disease including glomerular endothelium dysfunction and lipohyalinosis, which are associated with vascular risk factors such as hypertension [56]. As the vascular supplies to the kidney and brain are similar, renal small vessel disease may also be indicative of the presence of small vessel disease in the brain [57].

Kidney and Cognitive Impairment

CKD is emerging as an independent risk factor for cognitive impairment [58–64].

There is a growing awareness that vascular dementia and degenerative dementia such as Alzheimer's disease share similar mechanisms and lesions [65–67]. There is the possibility that factors other than small vessel disease such as

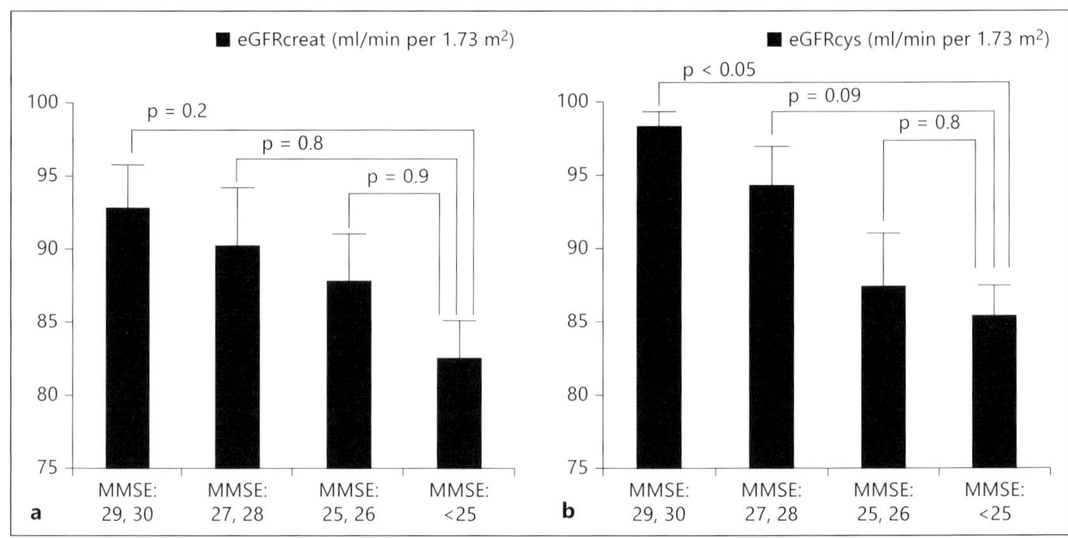

Fig. 4. Mean value of eGFR. Mean eGFR was presented according to the quartile of MMSE score. ANOVA was used to determine differences in eGFRcreat (**a**) and eGFRcys (**b**) among 4 groups. From Nagai and Kario [68].

Alzheimer's disease are involved in the pathogenesis of cognitive impairment in CKD. In fact, cystatin C, an innovative measure of kidney function, is reported to colocalize with β-amyloid in the brains of patients with Alzheimer's disease [66].

In the 3SCO study [68], we investigated the relationship between kidney function and cognitive function among 201 elderly at high risk of CVD. Kidney function was estimated based on serum creatinin (eGFRcreat) from the MDRD equation, and eGFR by CysC (eGFRcys) from Hoek's equation. Mean eGFRcreat and eGFRcys were 88.9 and 92.4 ml/min/1.73 m^2, respectively. In the analysis of variance, eGFRcreat showed no significant differences among the four quartiles of MMSE score (fig. 4a), while eGFRcys did ($p < 0.05$) (fig. 4b); specifically, the lowest MMSE score group had significantly lower eGFRcys than the highest MMSE score group ($p < 0.05$). In the high-risk elderly, eGFRcys was more closely associated with cognitive function than eGFRcreat.

Recently, Yamamoto et al. [69] investigated the relationships among kidney function, ABP measures, silent cerebral injury, and cognitive function in 224 patients with symptomatic lacunar infarction. Nondipper status, riser status, eGFR <60, and moderate-to-severe WMH were independently significantly associated with cognitive impairment. Higher age and eGFR <60 had significant associations with severe WML. Thus, nondipper and riser status and CKD seem to have a causal link with cognitive impairment.

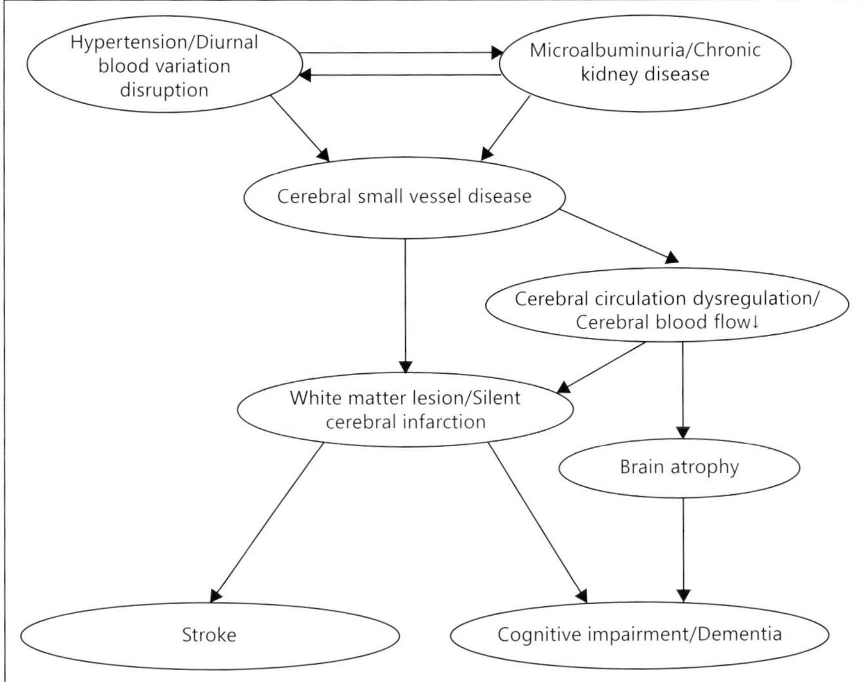

Fig. 5. Chart for the common pathophysiology for cerebral small vessel disease and stroke. Hypertension and impairment of kidney function are associated with each other. This relationship is suggested as a risk factor for cerebral small vessel disease, leading to both stroke and cognitive impairment.

Although there have been a few reports assessing the relationship among ABP, CKD, and target brain damage, nondipping status and CKD might each be independently associated with cognitive impairment.

Role of 24-Hour Blood Pressure Management in Preventing Kidney Disease and Stroke

Until now, there have been few reports assessing the relationship among 24-hour BP, CKD and stroke. Thus, it was not clear whether there was an interaction between high ABP and CKD for the stroke incidence. However, there is growing evidence that both high ABP and CKD were associated with cerebral small vessel disease and cognitive impairment. In these points, we focused on the relationships among diurnal BP variation disruption, CKD, and cerebral small vessel disease, and considered the factors shared in common by stroke and cognitive impairment (fig. 5). Active hypertensive treatment has been reported to be associated with reduced risks of microalbuminuria [70], WMH progression [42], and cognitive decline [67]. Thus, strict 24-hour BP control may be necessary to prevent the progression of kidney dysfunction, cognitive impairment, and stroke.

Conclusion

The recent literature confirms that both hypertension and CKD are associated with stroke. Also, the nondipping pattern and decreased kidney function have been found to be closely related with each other. Cerebral small vessel disease is considered to serve as a common pathophysiology in the relationship of hypertension and CKD with cognitive impairment and stroke. Strict 24-hour BP control during 24-hour may be necessary to prevent the progression of kidney dysfunction, cognitive impairment, and stroke.

Acknowledgements

The authors would like to acknowledge that this study was supported by a Research Grant for Geriatrics and Gerontology (22–5) from the Ministry of Health, Labor, and Welfare, Japan.

References

1 AHA: Heart Disease and Stroke Statistics – Update. 2005.
2 Wannamethee SG, Shaper AG, Perry IJ: Serum creatinine concentration and risk of cardiovascular disease: a possible marker for increased risk of stroke. Stroke 1997;28: 557–563.
3 Shlipak MG, Sarnak MJ, Katz R, Fried LF, Seliger SL, Newman AB, Siscovick DS, Stehman-Breen C: Cystatin C and the risk of death and cardiovascular events among elderly persons. N Engl J Med 2005;352:2049–2060.
4 Go AS, Chertow GM, Fan D, McCulloch CE, Hsu CY: Chronic kidney disease and the risks of death, cardiovascular events, and hospitalization. N Engl J Med 2004;351:1296–1305.
5 Pickering TG: Ambulatory blood pressure monitoring. Curr Hypertens Rep 2000;2:558–564.
6 Liao D, Cooper L, Cai J, Toole J, Bryan N, Burke G, Shahar E, Nieto J, Mosley T, Heiss G: The prevalence and severity of white matter lesions, their relationship with age, ethnicity, gender, and cardiovascular disease risk factors: the ARIC Study. Neuroepidemiology 1997;16:149–162.
7 Vermeer SE, Hollander M, van Dijk EJ, Hofman A, Koudstaal PJ, Breteler MM: Silent brain infarcts and white matter lesions increase stroke risk in the general population: the Rotterdam Scan Study. Stroke 2003;34: 1126–1129.
8 Chimowitz MI, Estes ML, Furlan AJ, Awad IA: Further observations on the pathology of subcortical lesions identified on magnetic resonance imaging. Arch Neurol 1992;49: 747–752.

9 Longstreth WT Jr, Manolio TA, Arnold A, Burke GL, Bryan N, Jungreis CA: Enright PL, O'Leary D, Fried L: Clinical correlates of white matter findings on cranial magnetic resonance imaging of 3,301 elderly people: the Cardiovascular Health Study. Stroke 1996;27:1274–1282.
10 Khatri M, Wright CB, Nickolas TL, Yoshita M, Paik MC, Kranwinkel G, Sacco RL, De-Carli C: Chronic kidney disease is associated with white matter hyperintensity volume: the Northern Manhattan Study (NOMAS). Stroke 2007;38:3121–3126.
11 Vupputuri S, Batuman V, Muntner P, Bazzano LA, Lefante JJ, Whelton PK, He J: Effect of blood pressure on early decline in kidney function among hypertensive men. Hypertension 2003;42:1144–1149.
12 Ninomiya T, Kiyohara Y, Tokuda Y, Doi Y, Arima H, Harada A, Ohashi Y, Ueshima H: Impact of kidney disease and blood pressure on the development of cardiovascular disease: an overview from the Japan Arteriosclerosis Longitudinal Study. Circulation 2008;118: 2694–2701.
13 Kokubo Y, Nakamura S, Okamura T, Yoshimasa Y, Makino H, Watanabe M, Higashiyama A, Kamide K, Kawanishi K, Okayama A, Kawano Y: Relationship between blood pressure category and incidence of stroke and myocardial infarction in an urban Japanese population with and without chronic kidney disease: the Suita Study. Stroke 2009;40: 2674–2679.
14 Kimura G: Kidney and circadian blood pressure rhythm. Hypertension 2008;51:827–828.
15 Lurbe E, Redon J, Kesani A, Pascual JM, Tacons J, Alvarez V, Batlle D: Increase in nocturnal blood pressure and progression to microalbuminuria in type 1 diabetes. N Engl J Med 2002;347:797–805.
16 Kimura G: Sodium, kidney, and circadian rhythm of blood pressure. Clin Exp Nephrol 2001;5:13–18.
17 Fukuda M, Munemura M, Usami T, Nakao N, Takeuchi O, Kamiya Y, Yoshida A, Kimura G: Nocturnal blood pressure is elevated with natriuresis and proteinuria as renal function deteriorates in nephropathy. Kidney Int 2004;65:621–625.
18 Rodgers A, MacMahon S, Gamble G, Slattery J, Sandercock P, Warlow C, UKTIA Collaborative Group: Blood pressure and risk of stroke in patients with cerebrovascular disease. BMJ 1996;313:147.
19 MacMahon S, Peto R, Cutler J, Collins R, Sorlie P, Neaton J, Abbott R, Godwin J, Dyer A, Stamler J: Blood pressure, stroke, and coronary heart disease. 1. Prolonged differences in blood pressure: prospective observational studies corrected for the regression dilution bias. Lancet 1990;335:765–774.
20 Rothwell PM, Howard SC, Dolan E, O'Brien E, Dobson JE, Dahlof B, Sever PS, Poulter NR: Prognostic significance of visit-to-visit variability, maximum systolic blood pressure, and episodic hypertension. Lancet 2010;375: 938–948.
21 Nagai M, Hoshide S, Ishikawa J, Shimada K, Kario K: Visit-to-visit blood pressure variations: new independent determinants for carotid artery measures in the elderly at high risk of cardiovascular disease. J Am Soc Hypertens 2011;5:184–192.
22 Brickman AM, Reitz C, Luchsinger JA, Manly JJ, Schupf N, Muraskin J, DeCarli C, Brown TR, Mayeux R: Long-term blood pressure fluctuation and cerebrovascular disease in an elderly cohort. Arch Neurol 2010;67: 564–569.
23 Skoog I, Lernfelt B, Landahl S, Palmertz B, Andreasson LA, Nilsson L, Persson G, Oden A, Svanborg A: 15-year longitudinal study of blood pressure and dementia. Lancet 1996; 347:1141–1145.
24 Stewart R, Xue QL, Masaki K, Petrovitch H, Ross GW, White LR, Launer LJ: Change in blood pressure and incident dementia: a 32-year prospective study. Hypertension 2009; 54:233–240.
25 McGuinness B, Todd S, Passmore P, Bullock R: The effects of blood pressure lowering on development of cognitive impairment and dementia in patients without apparent prior cerebrovascular disease. Cochrane Database Syst Rev 2006;2:CD004034.

26 Peters R, Beckett N, Forette F, Tuomilehto J, Clarke R, Ritchie C, Waldman A, Walton A, Poulter R, Ma S, Comsa M, Burch L, Fletcher A, Bulpitt C, HYVET Investigators: Incident dementia and blood pressure lowering in the Hypertension in the Very Elderly Trial cognitive function assessment (HYVET-COG): a double-blind, placebo controlled trial. Lancet Neurol 2008;7:683–689.
27 Fournier A, Oprisiu-Fournier R, Serot JM, Godefroy O, Achard JM, Faure S, Mazouz H, Temmer M, Albu A, Bordet R, Hanon O, Gueyffier F, Wang J, Black S, Sato N: Prevention of dementia by antihypertensive drugs: how AT1-receptor-blockers and dihydropyridines better prevent dementia in hypertensive patients than thiazides and ACE-inhibitors. Expert Rev Neurother 2009;9:1413–1431.
28 Qiu C, von Strauss E, Winblad B, Fratiglioni L: Decline in blood pressure over time and risk of dementia: a longitudinal study from the Kungsholmen project. Stroke 2004;35: 1810–1815.
29 Sakakura K, Ishikawa J, Okuno M, Shimada K, Kario K: Exaggerated ambulatory blood pressure variability is associated with cognitive function in the very elderly and quality of life in the younger elderly. Am J Hypertens 2007;20:720–727.
30 Nagai M, Hoshide S, Ishikawa J, Shimada K, Kario K: Visit-to-visit blood pressure variations: new independent determinants for cognitive function in the elderly at high risk of cardiovascular disease. J Hypertens 2012; 30:1556–1563.
31 Kario K, Pickering TG, Matsuo T, Hoshide S, Schwartz JE, Shimada K: Stroke prognosis and abnormal nocturnal blood pressure falls in older hypertensives. Hypertension 2001; 38:852–857.
32 Kario K, Shimada K, Schwartz JE, Matsuo T, Hoshide S, Pickering TG: Silent and clinically overt stroke in older Japanese subjects with white-coat and sustained hypertension. J Am Coll Cardiol 2001;38:238–245.
33 Shimada K, Kawamoto A, Matsubayashi K, Nishinaga M, Kimura S, Ozawa T: Diurnal blood pressure variations and silent cerebrovascular damage in elderly patients with hypertension. J Hypertens 1992;10:875–878.
34 Kario K, Matsuo T, Kobayashi H, Imiya M, Matsuo M, Shimada K: Nocturnal fall of blood pressure and silent cerebrovascular damage in elderly hypertensive patients. Advanced silent cerebrovascular damage in extreme dippers. Hypertension 1996;27:130–135.
35 Kario K, Pickering TG, Umeda Y, Hoshide S, Hoshide Y, Morinari M, Murata M, Kuroda T, Schwartz JE, Shimada K: Morning surge in blood pressure as a predictor of silent and clinical cerebrovascular disease in elderly hypertensives: a prospective study. Circulation 2003;107:1401–1406.
36 Tohgi H, Chiba K, Kimura M: Twenty-four-hour variation of blood pressure in vascular dementia of the Binswanger type. Stroke 1991;22:603–608.
37 Puisieux F, Monaca P, Deplanque D, Delmaire C, di Pompeo C, Monaca C, Leys D, Pruvo JP, Dewailly P: Relationship between leuko-araiosis and blood pressure variability in the elderly. Eur Neurol 2001;46 :115–120.
38 Nagai M, Hoshide S, Kario K: Association of prothrombotic status with markers of cerebral small vessel disease in elderly hypertensive patients. Am J Hypertens 2012;25:1088–1094.
39 Schwartz GL, Bailey KR, Mosley T, Knopman DS, Jack CR Jr, Canzanello VJ, Turner ST: Association of ambulatory blood pressure with ischemic brain injury. Hypertension 2007;49:1228–1234.
40 Birns J, Morris R, Jarosz J, Markus H, Kalra L: Ethnic differences in the cerebrovascular impact of hypertension. Cerebrovasc Dis 2008;25:408–416.
41 White WB, Wolfson L, Wakefield DB, Hall CB, Campbell P, Moscufo N, Schmidt J, Kaplan RF, Pearlson G, Guttman CR: Average daily blood pressure, not office blood pressure, is associated with progression of cerebrovascular disease and cognitive decline in older people. Circulation 2011;124:2312–2319.
42 Godin O, Tzourio C, Maillard P, Mazoyer B, Dufouil C: Antihypertensive treatment and change in blood pressure are associated with the progression of white matter lesion volumes: the Three-City (3C)-Dijon Magnetic Imaging Study. Circulation 2011;123:266–273.

43 Salerno JA, Murphy DG, Horwitz B, DeCarli C, Haxby JV, Rapoport SI, Schapiro MB: Brain atrophy in hypertension. A volumetric magnetic resonance imaging study. Hypertension 1992;20:340–348.

44 Goldstein IB, Bartzokis G, Guthrie D, Shapiro D: Ambulatory blood pressure and brain atrophy in the healthy elderly. Neurology 2002;59:713–719.

45 Nagai M, Hoshide S, Ishikawa J, Shimada K, Kario K: Ambulatory blood pressure as an independent determinant of brain atrophy and cognitive function in elderly hypertension. J Hypertens 2008;26:1636–1641.

46 Hajjar I, Zhao P, Alsop D, Abduljalil A, Selim M, Novak P, Novak V: Association of blood pressure elevation and nocturnal dipping with brain atrophy in stroke and nonstroke individuals. Am J Hypertens 2010;23:17–23.

47 Nagai M, Kario K: Blood pressure, aging, vascular disease, and their effects on brain volume. Am J Hypertens 2009;22:1135.

48 Nagai M, Hoshide S, Kario K: Hypertension and dementia. Am J Hypertens 2010;23:116–124.

49 Fazekas G, Fazekas F, Schmidt R, Kapeller P, Offenbacher H, Krejs GJ: Brain MRI findings and cognitive impairment in patients undergoing chronic hemodialysis treatment. J Neurol Sci 1995;134:83–88.

50 Shlipak MG, Fried LF, Crump C, Bleyer AJ, Manolio TA, Tracy RP, Furberg CD, Psaty BM: Elevations of inflammatory and procoagulant biomarkers in elderly persons with renal insufficiency. Circulation 2003;107:87–92.

51 Stuveling EM, Hillege HL, Bakker SJ, Gans RO, De Jong PE, De Zeeuw D: C-reactive protein is associated with renal function abnormalities in a non-diabetic population. Kidney Int 2003;63:654–661.

52 Wright CB, Paik MC, Brown TR, Stabler SP, Allen RH, Sacco RL, DeCarli C: Total homocysteine is associated with white matter hyperintensity volume: the Northern Manhattan Study. Stroke 2005;36:1207–1211.

53 Longstreth WT Jr, Arnold AM, Beauchamp NJ Jr, Manolio TA, Lefkowitz D, Jungreis C, Hirsch CH, O'Leary DH, Furberg CD: Incidence, manifestations, and predictors of worsening white matter on serial cranial magnetic resonance imaging in the elderly: the Cardiovascular Health Study. Stroke 2005;36:56–61.

54 Knopman DS, Mosley TH Jr, Bailey KR, Jack CR Jr, Schwartz GL, Turner ST: Associations of microalbuminuria with brain atrophy and white matter hyperintensities in hypertensive sibships. J Neurol Sci 2008;27:53–60.

55 Wiener DE, Bartolomei K, Scott T, Price LL, Griffith JL, Rosenberg I, Levey AS, Folstein MF, Sarnak MJ: Albuminuria, cognitive functioning, and white matter hyperintensities in homebound elders. Am J Kidney Dis 2009;53: 438–447.

56 Endemann DH, Schiffrin EL: Endothelial dysfunction. J Am Soc Nephrol 2004;15: 1983–1992.

57 Ito S, Nagasawa T, Abe M, Mori T: Strain vessel hypothesis: a viewpoint for linkage of albuminuria and cerebro-cardiovascular risk. Hypertens Res 2009;32:115–121.

58 Kurella Tamura M, Wadley V, Yaffe K, McClure LA, Howard G, Go R, Allman RM, Warnock DG, McClellan W: Kidney function and cognitive impairment in US adults: the Reasons for Geographic and Racial Differences in Stroke (REGARDS) Study. Am J Kidney Dis 2008;52:227–234.

59 Hailpern SM, Melamed ML, Cohen HW, Hostetter TH: Moderate chronic kidney disease and cognitive function in adults 20 to 59 years of age: Third National Health and Nutrition Examination Survey (NHANES III). J Am Soc Nephrol 2007;18:2205–2213.

60 Elias MF, Elias PK, Seliger SL, Narsipur SS, Dore GA, Robbins MA: Chronic kidney disease, creatinine and cognitive functioning. Nephrol Dial Transplant 2009;24:2446–2452.

61 Buchman AS, Tanne D, Boyle PA, Shah RC, Leurgans SE, Bennett DA: Kidney function is associated with the rate of cognitive decline in the elderly. Neurology 2009;73:920–927.

62 Etgen T, Sander D, Chonchol M, Briesenick C, Poppert H, Förstl H, Bickel H: Chronic kidney disease is associated with incident cognitive impairment in the elderly: the INVADE study. Nephrol Dial Transplant 2009; 24:3144–3150.

63 Khatri M, Nickolas T, Moon YP, Paik MC, Rundek T, Elkind MS, Sacco RL, Wright CB: CKD associates with cognitive decline. J Am Soc Nephrol 2009;20:2427–2432.

64 Tsai CF, Wang SJ, Fuh JL: Moderate chronic kidney disease is associated with reduced cognitive performance in midlife women. Kidney Int 2010;78:605–610.

65 Sinka L, Kövari E, Gold G, Hof PR, Herrmann FR, Bouras C, Giannakopoulos P: Small vascular and Alzheimer disease-related pathologic determinants of dementia in the oldest-old. J Neuropathol Exp Neurol 2010; 69:1247–1255.
66 Gold G, Giannakopoulos P, Herrmann FR, Bouras C, Kövari E: Identification of Alzheimer and vascular lesion thresholds for mixed dementia. Brain 2007;130:2830–2836.
67 Forette F, Seux ML, Staessen JA, Thijs L, Babarskiene MR, Babeanu S, Bossini A, Fagard R, Gil-Extremera B, Laks T, Kobalava Z, Sarti C, Tuomilehto J, Vanhanen H, Webster J, Yodfat Y, Birkenhäger WH: The prevention of dementia with antihypertensive treatment: new evidence from the Systolic Hypertension in Europe (Syst-Eur) study. Systolic Hypertension in Europe Investigators. Arch Intern Med 2002;162:2046–2052.
68 Nagai M, Kario K: Chronic kidney disease, 24-h blood pressure burden and their effects of silent cerebral injury and cognitive impairment: might age serve as a modulator? Hypertens Res 2011;34;1253–1254.
69 Yamamoto Y, Ohara T, Nagakane Y, Tanaka E, Morii F, Koizumi T, Akiguchi I: Chronic kidney disease, 24-hour blood pressure and small vessel diseases are independently associated with cognitive impairment in lacunar infarct patients. Hypertens Res 2011;34:1276–1282.
70 Ruggenenti P, Fassi A, Ilieva AP, Bruno S, Iliev IP, Brusegan V, Rubis N, Gherardi G, Arnoldi F, Ganeva M, Ene-lordache B, Gaspari F, Perna A, Bossi A, Trevisan R, Dodesini AR, Remuzzi G, Bergamo Nephrologic Diabetes Complications Trial (BENEDICT) Investigators: Preventing microalbuminuria in type 2 diabetes. N Engl J Med 2004;351: 1941–1951.

Kazuomi Kario, MD, PhD, FACP, FACC, FAHA
Division of Cardiovascular Medicine, Department of Medicine
Jichi Medical University School of Medicine, Yakushiji 3311-1
Shimotsuke, Tochigi 329-0498 (Japan)
E-Mail kkario@jichi.ac.jp

Primary Prevention of Stroke in Kidney Disease

Toyoda K (ed): Brain, Stroke and Kidney.
Contrib Nephrol. Basel, Karger, 2013, vol 179, pp 81–91 (DOI: 10.1159/000346726)

Preventing Stroke and Systemic Embolism in Renal Patients with Atrial Fibrillation: Focus on Anticoagulation

Yousif Ahmad · Gregory Y.H. Lip

University of Birmingham Centre for Cardiovascular Sciences, City Hospital, Birmingham, UK

Abstract

Chronic kidney disease and atrial fibrillation (AF) commonly coexist, and data suggest that renal patients have AF rates in excess of double that encountered in the general population. These patients are at increased risk of stroke, regardless of the presence or absence of AF. Furthermore, a lower GFR causes increased thromboembolic risk in patients with AF – independent of other risk factors. The dilemma facing clinicians treating this cohort of patients is that renal insufficiency confers both a thromboembolic and a bleeding risk. Renal disease also commonly coexists with other risk factors for stroke and bleeding such as hypertension and advanced age. Furthermore, bleeding risk tracks stroke risk and many risk factors are common to both thromboembolism and haemorrhage. Patients with severe renal impairment are also actively excluded from the majority of trials for stroke prevention in AF, including those trials which informed the development of stroke risk factor scoring schemes. Therefore, patients with renal disease and AF present a unique management challenge. The available data suggests that the benefit from warfarin in terms of stroke reduction is not as clear as in the general population, and there is an increased risk of bleeding complications and even ectopic vascular calcification. Thus, it is problematic to extrapolate the benefits of warfarin in the general population to a subgroup that has been actively excluded from clinical trials. The new oral anticoagulants have relatively little data in patients with severe renal impairment, and all have an element of renal excretion. There is a need for large randomised control trials in patients with renal insufficiency and on haemodialysis to provide a bank of high-quality scientific data on which clinicians can base their management decisions. Until then, we must adopt a pragmatic approach which involves careful consideration of the relative risk of stroke and bleeding in each individual patient.

Chronic kidney disease and atrial fibrillation (AF) commonly coexist [1]. For example, the large Chronic Renal Insufficiency Cohort (CRIC) study group demonstrated that 1 in 5 of their patients had evidence of AF [2], which is a figure in excess of double that reported in the general population. The mechanisms by which renal failure leads to AF are not fully understood but they likely include the increased likelihood of hypertension, fluctuating electrolyte levels, fluid overload, pathological activation of the renin-angiotensin-aldosterone system and sympathetic nervous system activation. These patients with renal insufficiency are at increased risk of stroke, regardless of the presence or absence of AF [3]. Furthermore, it would appear that a lower GFR causes increased thromboembolic risk in patients with AF – independent of other known risk factors [4].

The patient with AF and chronic renal impairment represents a formidable clinical conundrum for the physician. As well as their increased stroke risk, these patients also have a very high risk for other cardiovascular events and mortality [5]. Significantly, when it comes to the decision of antithrombotic therapy for stroke prevention, these patients are also at substantially increased risk of bleeding [1]. This bleeding risk is even more pronounced in patients treated with oral anticoagulation [6].

Stroke and Bleeding Risk

Antithrombotic therapy to prevent stroke is the most important management consideration in AF, and contemporary guidelines [7] recommend a risk factor-based approach to this decision. The favoured risk scheme is the CHA_2DS_2-VASc score (table 1) [8] which has several advantages over the more limited $CHADS_2$ score [9]. It has been shown in various independent validation cohorts to reliably identify ‘truly low-risk patients’ (annual stroke rate <1%/year) and classes fewer patients as ‘intermediate’ risk than $CHADS_2$. It also seems to be at least as good as – or possibly better – than the $CHADS_2$ score at identifying high-risk patients [10]. As the most feared complication of antithrombotic therapy, bleeding risk can limit the use of anticoagulants [11]. The HAS-BLED score (table 2) [12] has been recommended by the ESC as a simple and effective way for clinicians to assess a patient’s bleeding risk. Abnormal renal function forms a part of this scoring scheme, and clinicians are prompted to consider correctable risk factors for bleeding (erratic INRs, concomitant NSAID or aspirin therapy, poorly controlled blood pressure). The HAS-BLED score has been validated in various large real-world cohorts [13], performing favourably when compared to other bleeding risk scores [14].

Table 1. The CHA2DS2-VASc score for risk of stroke in nonvalvular AF

Risk factor	Score
Congestive cardiac failure	1
Hypertension	1
Age ≥75	2
Diabetes mellitus	1
Stroke/TIA/thromboembolism	1
Vascular disease	1
Age 65–74	1
Sex category (female)	1
Maximum score	9

Congestive cardiac failure is defined as left ventricular ejection fraction ≤40%. Hypertension is defined as blood pressure consistently above 140/90 mm Hg or treated hypertension on medication. Vascular disease is defined as previous myocardial infarction, peripheral arterial disease or aortic plaque.

Table 2. The HAS-BLED score for bleeding risk

Risk factor	Score
Hypertension	1
Abnormal renal/liver function	1 or 2
Stroke	1
Bleeding tendency	1
Labile INR	1
Elderly (eg age>65, frail condition)	1
Drugs (concomitant aspirin, NSAIDs, etc) or alcohol abuse or excess	1 or 2
Maximum score	9

A score of 0–2 indicates low risk of bleeding; ≥3 indicates high risk of bleeding. Hypertension is defined as a systolic blood pressure >160 mm Hg. 1 point is awarded for each of abnormal renal or liver function, and drugs or alcohol.

Considerations in Renal Disease Patients

The dilemma facing clinicians treating this cohort of patients is that renal insufficiency confers both a thromboembolic risk and a bleeding risk. Chronic renal disease also commonly coexists with other risk factors for stroke and bleeding such as hypertension and advanced age. Furthermore, bleeding risk tracks stroke risk and many risk factors are common to both thromboembolism and haemorrhage [15, 16]. Patients with severe renal impairment are also actively excluded from the majority of trials for stroke prevention in AF, including those trials which informed the development of stroke risk factor scoring schemes. This means there is a paucity of high-quality scientific data on which clinicians can base their management decisions. Therefore, patients with renal disease and AF present a unique management challenge.

A study by Chan et al. [17] examined the association between warfarin, clopidogrel or aspirin and new stroke, mortality, and hospitalization in a retrospective cohort analysis of 1,671 incident haemodialysis patients with pre-existing AF. The use of warfarin was associated with an increased risk of new stroke: HR 1.93, 95% CI 1.29–2.90. There was no associated increase in mortality or hospitalisation. This risk for new stroke was most evident in patients who had no INR monitoring in the first 90 days of dialysis: HR 2.79, 95% CI 1.65–4.70. It is also possible a substantial proportion of these strokes were haemorrhagic in nature, as nearly a third of patients who survived a stroke had their warfarin discontinued.

Similar findings were reported in a retrospective observation cohort study by Wizemann et al. [18] in the Dialysis Outcomes and Practice Patterns Study. In those aged over 75 years of age warfarin was associated with a statistically significant increase in strokes: HR 2.17, 95% CI 1.04–2.63; $p = 0.04$. This effect did not reach statistical significance for younger patients. It is important to emphasise that this study did not differentiate between ischaemic and haemorrhagic strokes.

In a systematic review of bleeding rates for haemodialysis patients on warfarin [19] it was found that major bleeding rates were twice as high with warfarin compared to heparin or no warfarin. This data is based on case series or observational cohort studies, and has not been adjusted for INR control. A retrospective analysis of 255 patients [20] found that major bleeding rates on warfarin were 3.1%, compared to 0.8% for those on no antithrombotic therapy. Aspirin conferred a major bleeding rate of 4.4% and the combination of warfarin and aspirin 6.3%. The majority of bleeding episodes were in the gastrointestinal tract. The relative risk of warfarin alone did not reach statistical significance.

In addition to the balance of thromboembolic and haemorrhagic risk, warfarin has also been associated with ectopic vascular calcification. A link has been established between oral anticoagulation with vitamin K antagonists and calcific uraemic arteriopathy [21]. The development of this condition heralds a poor prognosis [22] and is a potential further deterrent to the prescription of anticoagulation for these patients.

A review by Yang et al. [23] discouraged the routine use of warfarin for AF patients on haemodialysis, taking into account the increased risks of bleeding and vascular calcification. They also pointed out the unknown benefit on the prevention of ischaemic stroke, and the suggestion of the (albeit limited) evidence that warfarin may even increase the risk of ischaemic stroke in this patient population.

The decision of whether to treat renal patients with warfarin is clearly far from straightforward. It is problematic to extrapolate the benefits of warfarin in the general population to a subgroup that has been actively excluded from clinical trials. There is a need for large randomised trials to help inform management strategies for this fragile high-risk population.

How to Approach Stroke Prevention for Atrial Fibrillation Patients with Chronic Kidney Disease

A proposal (see Figure 2) suggested by Lip [24] is that patients with chronic kidney disease should receive warfarin only if their stroke risk is particularly high, as denoted by a CHA_2DS_2-VASc score of 2 or greater (in the general population oral anticoagulation would be indicated with a CHA_2DS_2-VASc score of 1 or greater). Informally, the 'little c' in CHA_2DS_2-VASc can be used to denote 'chronic kidney disease', giving an extra point to the score – although this approach requires validation in larger studies specifically 'real world' non-anticoagulated cohort studies with a broad spectrum of renal (dys)function. It would be important not use trial cohorts that have selected populations based on trial inclusion/exclusion criteria and be confounded by the particular trial intervention(s) (eg by anticoagulation therapy).

Renal disease scores one point on the HAS-BLED score. Patients identified at increased risk of bleeding with a HAS-BLED score of 3 or greater should be kept under regular and judicious review. A high HAS-BLED score per se is not a contraindication to anticoagulation (indeed, the net clinical benefit balancing stroke versus bleeding is still in favour of anticoagulation), but raises awareness of those patients at high risk and to address the potentially correctable risk factors for bleeding (e.g. uncontrolled blood pressure, concomitant aspirin use with warfarin). Also, tight control over INR should be sought, with a high time in therapeutic range and a consequent minimising of both thromboembolic and haemorrhagic complications [25].

New Oral Anticoagulants

The emergence of a number of new oral anticoagulants has provided safe and effective alternatives to warfarin and shifted the landscape of stroke prevention in AF (fig. 1). Dabigatran, rivaroxaban and apixaban are all at least partially cleared by the kidneys, and patients with severe renal impairment (creatinine

Before initiating treatment; drug and dose selection should be made in consideration of the renal function

Recheck renal function if there is any clinical suspicion of a decline: intercurrent infection, commencement of nephrotoxic medication, evidence of hypovolaemia or dehydration

No renal impairment: no routine monitoring required

Mild renal impairment: yearly assessment of renal function

Moderate renal impairment: 6-monthly assessment of renal function and dose adjustment as necessary

Severe renal impairment: drug withdrawal or dose adjustment as necessary

Fig. 1. When to assess renal function with new oral anticoagulants.

clearance ≤30 ml/min) were excluded from the large phase 3 trials evaluating these drugs (table 3).

Dabigatran is an oral direct thrombin inhibitor that was compared to warfarin in the RE-LY trial [26]. The drug is predominantly (80%) cleared renally and is contraindicated in those with severe renal impairment (creatinine clearance <30 ml/min). The reduced dose of 110 mg b.d. is advised in Europe for those with moderate renal impairment, although in the US this dose was rejected in favour of 75 mg [27] – a dose that has never been studied in a randomised control trial. Subgroup analyses in RE-LY showed that the rates of stroke proportionally increased in patients with mild and moderate renal impairment. The efficacy and safety of dabigatran were independent of renal function. Since impairment of renal function can exert an effect on the rates of stroke and bleeding with dabigatran and therefore clinicians must assess renal function before initiating treatment. Periodic reassessments should be undertaken in patients with renal insufficiency and whenever a decline in renal function is suspected (intercurrent infection, commencement of nephrotoxic drugs, hypovolaemia or dehydration). It is important to note that dabigatran is highly protein-bound and therefore removed by haemodialysis – rendering it unsuitable for the population of renal patients on dialysis.

Rivaroxaban is an oral factor Xa inhibitor which was compared to warfarin in the ROCKET-AF trial [28]. Although predominantly metabolised by the liver, one third of the drug is still cleared renally. Again, patients with severe renal impairment (eGFR <30 ml/min) were excluded from this trial. Patients with moderate renal impairment (eGFR 30–49 ml/min) the dose was reduced to 15 mg o.d. A subgroup analysis of ROCKET-AF [29] reported on these patients, and found that CKD patients had a higher rate of stroke and embolism irrespective of which treatment they received. The benefits of rivaroxaban in patients with

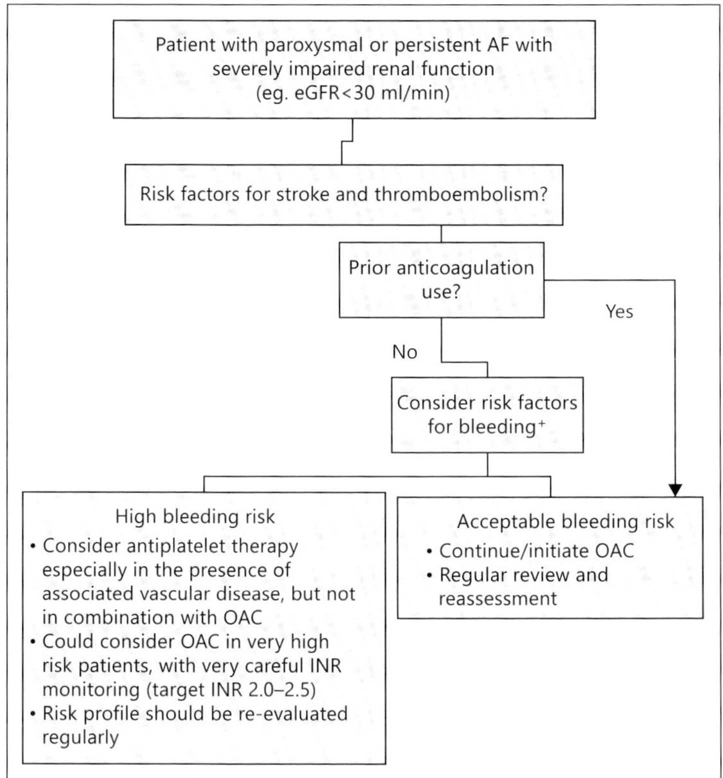

Fig. 2. Algorithm for oral anticoagulation therapy for stroke prevention in patients with atrial fibrillation and chronic renal disease [24]. Oral anticoagulation (OAC), for example, with vitamin K antagonists (VKAs, target INR 2–2.5) but new drugs which may be viable alternatives to the VKAs could ultimately be considered. Asterisk (*) signifies that risk factors for stroke and thromboembolism could be assessed using the CHA_2DS_2-VASc score, although the real stroke risk is likely to be much higher than reported in cohorts with no renal failure. If patients have already been taking OAC (e.g. for >3 months) with no bleeding complications, these patients probably represent a patient group that would 'tolerate' OAC with a lower bleeding risk. Plus (+) signifies that bleeding risk could be assessed using a validated scoring system (e.g. the HAS-BLED score) although the real bleeding risk may be higher than that reported in cohorts with no renal failure. A HAS-BLED score of ≥3 indicates the need for caution and/or regular review of the patient.

reduced renal function were consistent with those of the overall study population. There was not a significant payoff in terms of bleeding risk. Bleeding was not reported excessively with rivaroxaban than warfarin; there were fewer fatal bleeds with rivaroxaban (0.28 vs. 0.74% per 100 patient-years; $p = 0.047$). Interestingly, the rates of intracranial haemorrhage were similar between rivaroxaban and warfarin (0.71 vs. 0.88 per 100 patient-years; $p = 0.54$), meaning that im-

Table 3. Pharmacokinetic and pharmacodynamics properties of the novel anticoagulants

Mechanism of action	Direct thrombin inhibitor	Direct factor Xa inhibitor	Direct factor Xa inhibitor
Prodrug	double prodrug	no	no
Dosing frequency	twice daily	once daily	twice daily
Bioavailability, %	6.5	50	80
T_{max}	2 h	2–4 h	3 h
Half-life	17 h with multiple doses 7–9 h with single doses	9 h in healthy subjects 12 h in elderly subjects	12 h
Mode of excretion	80% cleared renally	one-third cleared renally, two-thirds metabolised by the liver	70% cleared in faeces 25% cleared renally
Age effect	affects pharmacokinetic parameters	no	no
Drug interactions	interaction with aspirin at high doses	none reported	none reported

paired renal function may obliterate rivaroxaban's benefit in terms of reducing intracranial haemorrhage.

Apixaban is another factor Xa inhibitor which was compared to warfarin in the ARISTOTLE trial [30]. The predominant route of clearance is through faeces, although 25% is still cleared by the kidneys. In keeping with the other trials, patients with severe renal insufficiency were excluded (creatinine clearance <25 ml/min). Once again, patients with renal impairment encountered more thromboembolic events than those with normal renal function. The reduction in the primary outcome of stroke or systemic embolism was consistent in patients with renal impairment compared to the rest of the study population. Of note, those patients with renal impairment (creatinine clearance 25–50 ml/min) received an increased benefit from apixaban in terms of reduction in major bleeding ($p = 0.03$ for interaction).

Conclusion

Despite the emergence of new anticoagulants which are safe and effective in the general AF population, clinicians still face a substantial challenge when treating patients with impaired renal function. These patients are often actively excluded from randomised control trials of new therapeutic agents. Furthermore, the data which forms the basis of risk stratification for both thromboembolism and bleeding in AF has not been validated in a population of patients with renal impairment. It is therefore difficult to assume that renal patients possess the same risk profile and will derive the same treatment benefits as the general population. There is a desperate need for large randomised control trials in patients with renal insufficiency and on haemodialysis to provide a bank of high-quality scientific data on which clinicians can base their management decisions. Until then, we must adopt a pragmatic approach which involved careful consideration of the relative risk of stroke and bleeding in each individual patient. These patients also warrant very close follow-up with excellent INR control for those on warfarin and judicious monitoring of renal function for those on a new drug.

References

1 Reinecke H, Brand E, Mesters R, Schäbitz WR, Fisher M, Pavenstädt H, Breithardt G: Dilemmas in the management of atrial fibrillation in chronic kidney disease. J Am Soc Nephrol 2009;20:705–711.

2 Soliman EZ, Prineas RJ, Go AS, Xie D, Lash JP, Rahman M, Ojo A, Teal VL, Jensvold NG, Robinson NL, Dries DL, Bazzano L, Mohler ER, Wright JT, Feldman HI, Chronic Renal Insufficiency Cohort (CRIC) Study Group: Chronic kidney disease and prevalent atrial fibrillation: the Chronic Renal Insufficiency Cohort (CRIC). Am Heart J 2010;159:1102–1107.

3 Lee M, Saver JL, Chang KH, Liao HW, Chang SC, Ovbiagele B: Low glomerular filtration rate and risk of stroke: meta-analysis. BMJ 2010;341:c4249.

4 Go AS, Fang MC, Udaltsova N, Chang Y, Pomernacki NK, Borowsky L, Singer DE, ATRIA Study Investigators: Impact of proteinuria and glomerular filtration rate on risk of thromboembolism in atrial fibrillation: the anticoagulation and risk factors in atrial fibrillation (ATRIA) study. Circulation 2009;119:1363–1369.

5 Di Angelantonio E, Chowdhury R, Sarwar N, Aspelund T, Danesh J, Gudnason V: Chronic kidney disease and risk of major cardiovascular disease and non-vascular mortality: prospective population based cohort study. BMJ 2010;341:c4986.

6 Chan KE, Lazarus JM, Thadhani R, Hakim RM: Warfarin use associates with increased risk for stroke in hemodialysis patients with atrial fibrillation. J Am Soc Nephrol 2009;20:2223–2233.

7 European Heart Rhythm Association, European Association for Cardio-Thoracic Surgery, Camm AJ, Kirchhof P, Lip GY, Schotten U, Savelieva I, Ernst S, Van Gelder IC, Al-Attar N, Hindricks G, Prendergast B, Heidbuchel H, Alfieri O, Angelini A, Atar D, Colonna P, De Caterina R, De Sutter J, Goette A, Gorenek B, Heldal M, Hohloser SH, Kolh P, Le Heuzey JY, Ponikowski P, Rutten FH: Guidelines for the management of atrial fibrillation: the Task Force for the Management of Atrial Fibrillation of the European Society of Cardiology (ESC). Eur Heart J 2010;31:2369–2429

8 Lip GY, Nieuwlaat R, Pisters R, Lane DA, Crijns HJ: Refining clinical risk stratification for predicting stroke and thromboembolism in atrial fibrillation using a novel risk factor-based approach: the euro heart survey on atrial fibrillation. Chest. 2010;137:263–272.

9 Karthikeyan G, Eikelboom JW: The CHADS2 score for stroke risk stratification in atrial fibrillation – friend or foe? Thromb Haemost 2010;104:45–48.

10 Van Staa TP, Setakis E, Di Tanna GL, Lane DA, Lip GY: A comparison of risk stratification schemes for stroke in 79,884 atrial fibrillation patients in general practice. J Thromb Haemost 2011;9:39–48.

11 Hylek EM, D'Antonio J, Evans-Molina C, Shea C, Henault LE, Regan S: Translating the results of randomized trials into clinical practice: the challenge of warfarin candidacy among hospitalized elderly patients with atrial fibrillation. Stroke 2006;37:1075–1080.

12 Lip GY, Andreotti F, Fauchier L, Huber K, Hylek E, Knight E, Lane D, Levi M, Marín F, Palareti G, Kirchhof P, European Heart Rhythm Association: Bleeding risk assessment and management in atrial fibrillation patients. Executive Summary of a Position Document from the European Heart Rhythm Association (EHRA), endorsed by the European Society of Cardiology (ESC) Working Group on Thrombosis. Thromb Haemost 2011;106:997–1011.
13 Olesen JB, Lip GY, Hansen PR, Lindhardsen J, Ahlehoff O, Andersson C, Weeke P, Hansen ML, Gislason GH, Torp-Pedersen C: Bleeding risk in 'real world' patients with atrial fibrillation: comparison of two established bleeding prediction schemes in a nationwide cohort. J Thromb Haemost 2011;9: 1460–1467.
14 Lip GY, Frison L, Halperin JL, Lane DA: Comparative validation of a novel risk score for predicting bleeding risk in anticoagulated patients with atrial fibrillation: the HAS-BLED (Hypertension, Abnormal Renal/Liver Function, Stroke, Bleeding History or Predisposition, Labile INR, Elderly, Drugs/Alcohol Concomitantly) score. J Am Coll Cardiol 2011;57:173–180.
15 Friberg L, Rosenqvist M, Lip GY: Net clinical benefit of warfarin in patients with atrial fibrillation: a report from the Swedish atrial fibrillation cohort study. Circulation 2012; 125:2298–2307.
16 Olesen JB, Lip GY, Lindhardsen J, Lane DA, Ahlehoff O, Hansen ML, Raunsø J, Tolstrup JS, Hansen PR, Gislason GH, Torp-Pedersen C: Risks of thromboembolism and bleeding with thromboprophylaxis in patients with atrial fibrillation: a net clinical benefit analysis using a 'real world' nationwide cohort study. Thromb Haemost 2011;106:739–749
17 Chan KE, Lazarus JM, Thadhani R, Hakim RM: Warfarin use associates with increased risk for stroke in hemodialysis patients with atrial fibrillation. J Am Soc Nephrol 2009;20: 2223–2233.
18 Wizemann V, Tong L, Satayathum S, Disney A, Akiba T, Fissell RB, Kerr PG, Young EW, Robinson BM: Atrial fibrillation in hemodialysis patients: clinical features and associations with anticoagulant therapy. Kidney Int 2010;77:1098–1106.
19 Elliott MJ, Zimmerman D, Holden RM: Warfarin anticoagulation in hemodialysis patients: a systematic review of bleeding rates. Am J Kidney Dis 2007;50:433–440.
20 Holden RM, Harman GJ, Wang M, Holland D, Day AG: Major bleeding in hemodialysis patients. Clin J Am Soc Nephrol 2008;3:105–110.
21 Streit M, Paredes BE, Rüegger S, Brand CU: Typical features of calciphylaxis in a patient with end-stage renal failure, diabetes mellitus and oral anticoagulation. Dermatology 2000; 200:356–359.
22 Fine A, Zacharias J: Calciphylaxis is usually non-ulcerating: risk factors, outcome and therapy. Kidney Int 2002;61:2210–2217.
23 Yang F, Chou D, Schweitzer P, Hanon S: Warfarin in haemodialysis patients with atrial fibrillation: what benefit? Europace 2010; 12:1666–1672.
24 Lip GY: Chronic renal disease and stroke in atrial fibrillation: balancing the prevention of thromboembolism and bleeding risk. Europace 2011;13:145–148.
25 Gallagher AM, Setakis E, Plumb JM, Clemens A, van Staa TP: Risks of stroke and mortality associated with suboptimal anticoagulation in atrial fibrillation patients. ThrombHaemost 2011;106:968–977.
26 Connolly SJ, Ezekowitz MD, Yusuf S, Eikelboom J, Oldgren J, Parekh A, Pogue J, Reilly PA, Themeles E, Varrone J, Wang S, Alings M, Xavier D, Zhu J, Diaz R, Lewis BS, Darius H, Diener HC, Joyner CD, Wallentin L, RE-LY Steering Committee and Investigators: Dabigatran versus warfarin in patients with atrial fibrillation. N Engl J Med 2009;361: 1139–1151.
27 Beasley BN, Unger EF, Temple R: Anticoagulant options – why the FDA approved a higher but not a lower dose of dabigatran. N Engl J Med 2011;364:1788–1790.
28 Patel MR, Mahaffey KW, Garg J, Pan G, Singer DE, Hacke W, Breithardt G, Halperin JL, Hankey GJ, Piccini JP, Becker RC, Nessel CC, Paolini JF, Berkowitz SD, Fox KA, Califf RM, ROCKET AF Investigators: Rivaroxaban versus warfarin in nonvalvular atrial fibrillation. N Engl J Med 2011;365:883–891.

29 Fox KA, Piccini JP, Wojdyla D, Becker RC, Halperin JL, Nessel CC, Paolini JF, Hankey GJ, Mahaffey KW, Patel MR, Singer DE, Califf RM: Prevention of stroke and systemic embolism with rivaroxaban compared with warfarin in patients with non-valvular atrial fibrillation and moderate renal impairment. Eur Heart J 2011;32:2387–2394.

30 Granger CB, Alexander JH, McMurray JJ, Lopes RD, Hylek EM, Hanna M, Al-Khalidi HR, Ansell J, Atar D, Avezum A, Bahit MC, Diaz R, Easton JD, Ezekowitz JA, Flaker G, Garcia D, Geraldes M, Gersh BJ, Golitsyn S, Goto S, Hermosillo AG, Hohnloser SH, Horowitz J, Mohan P, Jansky P, Lewis BS, Lopez-Sendon JL, Pais P, Parkhomenko A, Verheugt FW, Zhu J, Wallentin L, ARISTOTLE Committees and Investigators: Apixaban versus warfarin in patients with atrial fibrillation. N Engl J Med 2011;365:981–992.

Gregory Y.H. Lip
University of Birmingham Centre for Cardiovascular Sciences, City Hospital
Dudley Road
B18 7QH Birmingham (UK)
E-Mail g.y.h.lip@bham.ac.uk

Toyoda K (ed): Brain, Stroke and Kidney.
Contrib Nephrol. Basel, Karger, 2013, vol 179, pp 92–99 (DOI: 10.1159/000346727)

Stroke Features and Management in Patients with Chronic Kidney Disease

Masahiro Kamouchi

Department of Medicine and Clinical Science, Graduate School of Medical Sciences, and Department of Nephrology, Hypertension and Strokology, Kyushu University Hospital, Fukuoka, Japan

Abstract

Chronic kidney disease (CKD) is an independent risk factor for cardiovascular diseases, including stroke. Patients with CKD are susceptible to ischemic as well as hemorrhagic stroke. The impairments in the small vessel vasculature, atherosclerotic changes of the large vessels, and coagulation abnormalities in CKD probably underlie the specific characteristics of stroke in these patients. The clinical outcomes, including the functional outcomes and short- as well as long-term mortality after stroke, are poor in patients with CKD. CKD is defined as a decreased glomerular filtration rate (GFR) and/or increased urine albumin excretion. A number of studies have shown that either or both of these two markers were significantly associated with poor functional outcomes and mortality after stroke. Recent studies have suggested that proteinuria/albuminuria is more deeply involved in the clinical outcomes than GFR. Although the mechanisms responsible for their association are currently unclear, glomerular barrier and/or filtration dysfunction are probably related to the small vessel diseases, hypercoagulability and inflammation, which may affect the clinical outcomes in CKD patients after stroke. The evidence for the most effective management of acute stroke in CKD patients is lacking, and thus, the current treatment for stroke is optimized for individual patients based on their background. Further studies are thus needed to elucidate the specific features of stroke and also the management of stroke in patients with CKD.

Chronic kidney disease (CKD) is an independent risk factor for cardiovascular diseases, including stroke. Recent studies have shown that the markers of CKD, a reduced glomerular filtration rate (GFR) and/or increased albumin excretion, are associated with the incidence of cardiovascular diseases. However, so far there have been few studies concerning the clinical features of stroke in patients with CKD. Stroke in patients under kidney replacement therapy may have unique characteristics which are induced by the specific treatments and end-stage kidney disease. In this chapter, we focus on the impact of an impaired kidney function, such as a decreased glomerular filtration rate and/or barrier function on the features of the stroke. The management of stroke in CKD patients is also discussed, although no optimal treatment protocol has yet been established.

Characteristics of Stroke in CKD Patients

Stroke Subtypes

Although patients with CKD have risk factors for stroke, CKD is an independent risk factor for ischemic, as well as hemorrhagic, stroke. In a population-based cohort study, the relative risk for ischemic stroke was 4.3–10.1 and that for hemorrhagic stroke was 4.1–6.7, respectively, in dialysis patients [1]. Even in the patients with a mild level of glomerular dysfunction, the risk for stroke appears to be increased. A recent study with 20,386 participants without previous stroke has revealed that the incidence of stroke symptoms increased in patients with a lower estimated GFR (eGFR) and a higher level of albuminuria [2].

The impact of CKD on the stroke subtype may be different depending on gender. In 539,287 Swedish men and women free of previous stroke, the hazard ratios of renal dysfunction for ischemic stroke were 1.09, 1.24 and 2.27 for those with a mildly, moderately and severely decreased GFR, respectively. This trend was observed in both genders. In contrast, hemorrhagic stroke was only related to renal dysfunction in females; 1.39, 1.70 and 3.46 for a mildly, moderately and severely decreased GFR [3]. In a study of 12,222 Japanese men and women living in four communities, CKD increased the risk of hemorrhagic stroke, especially for males, but that of ischemic stroke for females. In that study, it was concluded that the gender difference was due to the differences in the prevalence of alcohol drinkers [4]. Therefore, CKD may have a gender-specific association with ischemic and hemorrhagic stroke, but this may differ according to the presence of other risk factors or in different ethnic groups.

Subtypes of Ischemic Stroke

Atherosclerosis is progressive in CKD patients. The prevalence of intracranial artery calcification was shown to be high in acute ischemic stroke patients with a reduced GFR [5]. Another study reported that proteinuria was an independent risk factor for ischemic stroke due to thrombotic arterial occlusion in patients with non-insulin-dependent diabetes mellitus [6].

A reduced GFR and increased excretion of albumin are factors closely associated with increased permeability or vulnerability of the small vessels, indepen-

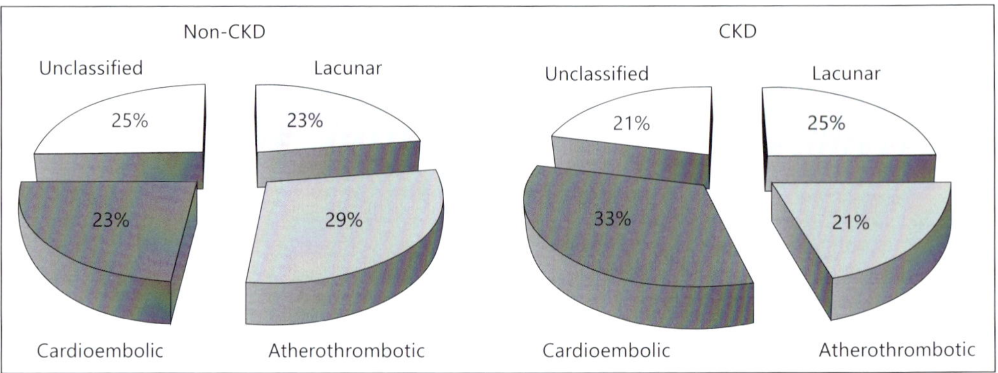

Fig. 1. Comparison of stroke subtypes in patients with and without CKD. Data were obtained from 10,642 patients with ischemic stroke enrolled in the Fukuoka Stroke Registry [Kamouchi et al., unpubl. data]. CKD was defined as a low eGFR (<60 ml/min/1.73 m^2).

dent of other risk factors. These changes are causative of white matter lesions, cerebral microbleeds and lacunar infarction. Recent studies showed that patients with a reduced GFR had more frequent lacunar strokes, as assessed by MRI [7]. Cerebral microbleeds were also shown to be associated with proteinuria [8], and with the level of microalbuminuria [9].

The prevalence of atrial fibrillation is high in patients with late-stage CKD, ranging from 7% to 27% in various studies [10]. The hypercoagulable state deteriorates in parallel with the severity of renal dysfunction. Go et al. [11] reported that in patients with atrial fibrillation, proteinuria and a lower eGFR increased the risk of thromboembolism, independent of other known risk factors. In our stroke database, cardioembolic stroke was more prevalent in patients with CKD than in those without (fig. 1).

Albuminuria or proteinuria is a surrogate for an increased permeability of the brain vasculature, and thus implies an increased susceptibility to hemorrhagic transformation after infarction. A recent study showed that albuminuria was an independent predictor for hemorrhagic transformation following acute ischemic stroke, even after adjustment for possible confounding factors. Albuminuria was shown to be associated with parenchymal hemorrhage [13].

Clinical Outcomes in Stroke Patients with CKD

Functional Outcomes

CKD is associated with the functional outcomes in patients with acute stoke [14]. Ovbiagele et al. [15] investigated the association between proteinuria or a low eGFR and functional activities in patients with an acute ischemic stroke without known CKD. They found that the clinical outcomes were poorer in relation to proteinuria, but not to a low GFR. Recently, our group also demonstrated that proteinuria, but not a reduced eGFR, was associated with a poor functional outcome after ischemic stroke [12]. It has been shown that in patients with lacunar stroke, the progression of neurological symptoms occurred more often in those with albuminuria. Albuminuria was an independent predictor of the neurological progression in patients with a lacunar stroke, and the progression was associated with a worse outcome at 90 days [16]. Slowik et al. [17] reported that patients with microalbuminuria showed a more severe neurological deficit and presented more decreased levels of consciousness (table 1).

In cases of hemorrhagic stroke, moderate-to-severe CKD was associated with a larger hematoma volume [18]. However, another study showed that, in patients with intracerebral hemorrhage, proteinuria and a low eGFR were not linked to the patient being discharged directly to home [19].

Mortality

A recent study showed that CKD was also significantly associated with in-hospital mortality after stroke, regardless of the stroke subtypes, ischemic stroke, intracerebral hemorrhage and subarachnoid hemorrhage. This association was more pronounced in patients with a younger age and in females [20]. A low GFR or proteinuria, or both, have been suggested to be involved in the short-term mortality after stroke. In patients with ischemic stroke, both proteinuria and a lower eGFR were predictive factors for the 30-day mortality [21]. We found that proteinuria, but not a reduced eGFR, was associated with the in-hospital mortality after acute ischemic stroke [12]. Slowik et al. [17] also reported microalbuminuria to be an independent predictor of the 1-year mortality. The long-term mortality after stroke for as long as 7 [22] or 10 years [23] was reported to be associated with a reduced GFR at baseline (table 2).

The mechanism by which CKD is associated with poor outcomes after stroke is unknown. Oksala et al. [24] reported that a reduced eGFR and cerebral small vessel diseases were associated with poststroke long-term survival. In patients with ischemic stroke, acute kidney injury tended to occur in those with a reduced GFR after acute stroke, and was associated with short-term survival. Since baseline renal function was an independent predictor for acute kidney injury, poor functional outcomes may be partially mediated by acute kidney injury [25, 26].

Table 1. Summary of the relationship between CKD and the functional outcomes after acute stroke

Study	Number of subjects	Follow-up	Stroke subtype	Indices of CKD	Clinical outcome	CKD and functional outcome
Slowik et al. [17]	60 first ever stroke, 50 recurrent stroke	30 days	ischemic stroke	microalbuminuria	neurological deficit (SSS)	more severe deficit
Ovbiagele et al. [15]	251	during hospitalization	TIA and ischemic stroke	eGFR <60 ml/min/1.73 m^2; proteinuria	poor functional outcome (mRS2-6); discharge to home	eGFR, no association; proteinuria, independent predictor
Yahalom et al. [14]	821	1 month, 1 year	stroke (ischemic stroke 86%)	eGFR <60 ml/min/1.73 m^2	poor functional outcome (BI ≤75 or death)	independent predictor
Agrawal et al. [27]	74	during hospitalization eGFR ≥60 ml/min/1.73 m^2,8 (5–10) days eGFR <60 ml/min/1.73 m^2,7 (4–14) days	ischemic stroke treated with t-PA	eGFR <60 ml/min/1.73 m^2	intracranial hemorrhage; poor functional outcome (mRS 3–6)	no association
Ovbiagele et al. [19]	94	during hospitalization	intracerebral hemorrhage	eGFR <60 ml/min/1.73 m^2; proteinuria	discharge to home	no association
Cuadrado-Godia et al. [16]	127	72 h	lacunar stroke	albuminuria	neurological worsening (NIHSS ≥4)	independent predictor
Naganuma et al. [28]	578	3 months	ischemic stroke treated with t-PA	eGFR <60 ml/min/1.73 m^2	poor functional outcome (mRS 4-6)	independent predictor
Kumai et al. [12]	3,778	during hospitalization	ischemic stroke	eGFR; proteinuria	neurological worsening (NIHSS ≥2); poor functional outcome (mRS 2–6)	eGFR, no association; proteinuria, independent predictor

SSS = Scandinavian Stroke Scale; eGFR = estimated glomerular filtration rate; mRS = modified Rankin scale; BI = Barthel index; t-PA = tissue plasminogen activator; NIHSS = National Institute of Health Stroke Scale.

Management of Acute Stroke in CKD Patients

Tissue-Plasminogen Activator

It still remains controversial as to whether tissue-plasminogen activator is beneficial or detrimental to the clinical outcomes after ischemic stroke complicated by CKD. Hemorrhagic infarction is a major concern after thrombolytic therapy in CKD patients, because hemorrhagic transformation or cerebral microbleeds are more prevalent in these patients. Agrawal et al. [27] reported that an eGFR <60 ml/min/1.73 m^2 was not associated with an increased risk of symptomatic intracra-

Table 2. Summary of the association between CKD and mortality after acute stroke

Study	Number of subjects	Stroke subtype	Indices of CKD	Clinical outcome	CKD and mortality
MacWalter et al. [22]	2,042	stroke	Ccr ≥51.27 ml/min serum Cr≥119 μmol/l serum urea ≥9 mmol/l urea/Cr ratio ≥0.08573 mol/μmol	7-year mortality	all indices, independent predictors
Slowik et al. [17]	60 first ever stroke, 50 recurrent stroke	ischemic stroke	microalbuminuria	1-year mortality	independent predictor
Tsagalis et al. [23]	1,193	stroke (ischemic stroke 85%)	eGFR<60 ml/min/ 1.73 m^2	10-year mortality	independent predictor
Brzosko et al. [21]	312	ischemic stroke	eGFR<60 ml/min/ 1.73 m^2 Proteinuria	30-day mortality	independent predictor
Yahalom et al. [14]	821	stroke (ischemic stroke 86%)	eGFR<60 ml/min/ 1.73 m^2	1-year mortality	independent predictor
Agrawal et al. [27]	74	ischemic stroke treated with t-PA	eGFR<60 ml/min/ 1.73 m^2	in-hospital mortality	no association
Oksala et al. [24]	378	ischemic stroke	eGFR<60 ml/min/ 1.73 m^2	12-year mortality	independent predictor
Ovbiagele et al. [20]	1,127,842	ischemic stroke, intracerebral hemorrhage, subarachnoid hemorrhage	CKD	in-hospital mortality	independent predictor
Naganuma et al. [28]	578	ischemic stroke treated with t-PA	eGFR<60 ml/min/ 1.73 m^2	3-month mortality	independent predictor
Kumai et al. [12]	3,778	ischemic stroke	eGFR; proteinuria	in-hospital mortality	eGFR, no association; proteinuria, independent predictor

C_{Cr} = Creatinine clearance; Cr = creatinine; eGFR = estimated glomerular filtration rate; t-PA = tissue plasminogen activator.

nial hemorrhage, poor functional outcomes or in-hospital death in patients receiving thrombolytic therapy. They concluded that the clinical outcomes after the use of thrombolytic therapy were similar between those with and without CKD. However, another recent study has shown contradictory results, thus suggesting that a reduced eGFR was associated with early intracerebral hemorrhage and poor outcomes after 3 months in patients treated with tissue-plasminogen activator [28].

Anticoagulation Therapy

In patients with CKD, a variety of factors, including the treatments being administered, affect the coagulation and fibrinolytic states, leading to thrombosis and/or hemorrhage. The use of warfarin is associated with an improved survival in dialysis patients with atrial fibrillation [29]. In high-risk patients with stage 3 CKD, an adjusted dose of warfarin was suggested to be effective to reduce the risk of ischemic stroke and systemic embolism [30]. Anticoagulation therapy with warfarin targeting an INR between 2.0 and 3.0 is probably effective in CKD patients with atrial fibrillation to reduce the risk of thromboembolic stroke without increasing major bleeding. However, the efficacy and optimal intensity of anticoagulation to prevent early recurrence after cardioembolic stroke in CKD patients with atrial fibrillation are currently unknown.

References

1 Seliger SL, Gillen DL, Longstreth WT Jr, Kestenbaum B, Stehman-Breen CO: Elevated risk of stroke among patients with end-stage renal disease. Kidney Int 2003;64:603–609.

2 Muntner P, Judd SE, McClellan W, Meschia JF, Warnock DG, Howard VJ: Incidence of stroke symptoms among adults with chronic kidney disease: results from the REasons for Geographic And Racial Differences in Stroke (REGARDS) study. Nephrol Dial Transplant 2012;27:166–173.

3 Holzmann MJ, Aastveit A, Hammar N, Jungner I, Walldius G, Holme I: Renal dysfunction increases the risk of ischemic and hemorrhagic stroke in the general population. Ann Med 2012;44:607–615.

4 Shimizu Y, Maeda K, Imano H, Ohira T, Kitamura A, Kiyama M, Okada T, Ishikawa Y, Shimamoto T, Yamagishi K, Tanigawa T, Iso H: Chronic kidney disease and drinking status in relation to risks of stroke and its subtypes. The Circulatory Risk in Communities Study (CIRCS). Stroke 2011;42:2531–2537.

5 Bugnicourt JM, Chillon JM, Massy ZA, Canaple S, Lamy C, Deramond H, Godefroy O: High prevalence of intracranial artery calcification in stroke patients with CKD: a retrospective study. Clin J Am Soc Nephrol 2009;4:284–290.

6 Guerrero-Romero F, Rodriguez-Moran M: Proteinuria is an independent risk factor for ischemic stroke in non-insulin-dependent diabetes mellitus. Stroke 1999;30:1787–1791.

7 Ikram MA, Vernooij MW, Hofman A, Niessen WJ, van der Lugt A, Breteler MM: Kidney function is related to cerebral small vessel disease. Stroke 2008;39:55–61.

8 Ovbiagele B, Liebeskind DS, Pineda S, Saver JL: Strong independent correlation of proteinuria with cerebral microbleeds in patients with stroke and transient ischemic attack. Arch Neurol 2010;67:45–50.

9 Umemura T, Kawamura T, Sakakibara T, Mashita S, Hotta N, Sobue G: Microalbuminuria is independently associated with deep or infratentorial brain microbleeds in hypertensive adults. Am J Hypertens 2012;25:430–436.

10 Aronow WS: Acute and chronic management of atrial fibrillation in patients with late-stage CKD. Am J Kidney Dis 2009;53:701–710.

11 Go AS, Fang MC, Udaltsova N, Chang Y, Pomernacki NK, Borowsky L, Singer DE: Impact of proteinuria and glomerular filtration rate on risk of thromboembolism in atrial fibrillation: the anticoagulation and risk factors in atrial fibrillation (ATRIA) study. Circulation 2009;119:1363–1369.

12 Kumai Y, Kamouchi M, Hata J, Ago T, Kitayama J, Nakane H, Sugimori H, Kitazono T: Proteinuria and clinical outcomes after ischemic stroke. Neurology 2012;78:1909–1915.

13 Rodriguez-Yanez M, Castellanos M, Blanco M, Millan M, Nombela F, Sobrino T, Lizasoain I, Leira R, Serena J, Davalos A, Castillo J: Micro- and macroalbuminuria predict hemorrhagic transformation in acute ischemic stroke. Neurology 2006;67:1172–1177.

14 Yahalom G, Schwartz R, Schwammenthal Y, Merzeliak O, Toashi M, Orion D, Sela BA, Tanne D: Chronic kidney disease and clinical outcome in patients with acute stroke. Stroke 2009;40:1296–1303.

15 Ovbiagele B, Sanossian N, Liebeskind DS, Kim D, Ali LK, Pineda S, Saver JL: Indices of kidney dysfunction and discharge outcomes in hospitalized stroke patients without known renal disease. Cerebrovasc Dis 2009; 28:582–588.
16 Cuadrado-Godia E, Ois A, Garcia-Ramallo E, Giralt E, Jimena S, Rubio MA, Rodriguez-Campello A, Jimenez-Conde J, Roquer J: Biomarkers to predict clinical progression in small vessel disease strokes: prognostic role of albuminuria and oxidized LDL cholesterol. Atherosclerosis 2011;219:368–372.
17 Slowik A, Turaj W, Iskra T, Strojny J, Szczudlik A: Microalbuminuria in nondiabetic patients with acute ischemic stroke: prevalence, clinical correlates, and prognostic significance. Cerebrovasc Dis 2002;14:15–21.
18 Molshatzki N, Orion D, Tsabari R, Schwammenthal Y, Merzeliak O, Toashi M, Tanne D: Chronic kidney disease in patients with acute intracerebral hemorrhage: Association with large hematoma volume and poor outcome. Cerebrovas Dis 2011;31:271–277.
19 Ovbiagele B, Pineda S, Saver JL: Renal dysfunction and discharge destination in patients with intracerebral hemorrhage. J Stroke Cerebrovasc Dis 2011;20:145–149.
20 Ovbiagele B: Chronic kidney disease and risk of death during hospitalization for stroke. J Neurol Sci 2011;301:46–50.
21 Brzosko S, Szkolka T, Mysliwiec M: Kidney disease is a negative predictor of 30-day survival after acute ischaemic stroke. Nephron Clin Pract 2009;112:c79–c85.
22 MacWalter RS, Wong SY, Wong KY, Stewart G, Fraser CG, Fraser HW, Ersoy Y, Ogston SA, Chen R: Does renal dysfunction predict mortality after acute stroke? A 7-year follow-up study. Stroke 2002;33:1630–1635.
23 Tsagalis G, Akrivos T, Alevizaki M, Manios E, Stamatellopoulos K, Laggouranis A, Vemmos KN: Renal dysfunction in acute stroke: an independent predictor of long-term all combined vascular events and overall mortality. Nephrol Dial Transplant 2009;24:194–200.
24 Oksala NK, Salonen T, Strandberg T, Oksala A, Pohjasvaara T, Kaste M, Karhunen PJ, Erkinjuntti T: Cerebral small vessel disease and kidney function predict long-term survival in patients with acute stroke. Stroke 2010;41:1914–1920.
25 Covic A, Schiller A, Mardare NG, Petrica L, Petrica M, Mihaescu A, Posta N: The impact of acute kidney injury on short-term survival in an Eastern European population with stroke. Nephrol Dial Transplant 2008;23: 2228–2234.
26 Tsagalis G, Akrivos T, Alevizaki M, Manios E, Theodorakis M, Laggouranis A, Vemmos KN: Long-term prognosis of acute kidney injury after first acute stroke. Clin J Am Soc Nephrol 2009;4:616–622.
27 Agrawal V, Rai B, Fellows J, McCullough PA: In-hospital outcomes with thrombolytic therapy in patients with renal dysfunction presenting with acute ischaemic stroke. Nephrol Dial Transplant 2010;25:1150–1157.
28 Naganuma M, Koga M, Shiokawa Y, Nakagawara J, Furui E, Kimura K, Yamagami H, Okada Y, Hasegawa Y, Kario K, Okuda S, Nishiyama K, Minematsu K, Toyoda K: Reduced estimated glomerular filtration rate is associated with stroke outcome after intravenous rt-PA. The Stroke Acute Management with Urgent Risk-Factor Assessment and Improvement (SAMURAI) rt-PA registry. Cerebrovasc Dis 2011;31:123–129.
29 Abbott KC, Trespalacios FC, Taylor AJ, Agodoa LY: Atrial fibrillation in chronic dialysis patients in the United States. Risk factors for hospitalization and mortality. BMC Nephrol 2003;4:1.
30 Hart RG, Pearce LA, Asinger RW, Herzog CA: Warfarin in atrial fibrillation patients with moderate chronic kidney disease. Clin J Am Soc Nephrol 2011;6:2599–2604.

Masahiro Kamouchi, MD, PhD
Department of Medicine and Clinical Science
Graduate School of Medical Sciences, Kyushu University
Maidashi 3-1-1, Higashi-ku, Fukuoka 812-8582 (Japan)
E-Mail kamouchi@intmed2.med.kyushu-u.ac.jp

Toyoda K (ed): Brain, Stroke and Kidney.
Contrib Nephrol. Basel, Karger, 2013, vol 179, pp 100–109 (DOI: 10.1159/000346728)

Stroke Feature and Management in Dialysis Patients

Kunitoshi Iseki

Dialysis Unit, University Hospital of the Ryukyus, Okinawa, Japan

Abstract

Strokes remain the major complication among dialysis population as the number of diabetes and elderly is increasing. In chronic hemodialysis patients, prevalence and incidence of stroke is higher than that of the general population. According to the annual registry data of the Japanese Society for Dialysis Therapy, prevalence of stroke death has been declining, yet the incidence of nonfatal incidence of stroke is not known. Underlying mechanisms of stroke are multiple. Among them, control of hypertension is important for the primary prevention; however, the ideal target level of blood pressure is not determined. Other than hypertension, maintaining good nutritional status is utmost important. Most observational studies suggested that the target was 140/90 mm Hg at prehemodialysis session. However, blood pressure levels are variable in both at office (before and after dialysis session) and at home. It is advisable to measure blood pressure multiple occasions and also at home. In case of acute cerebral hemorrhage, glycerol is indicated to prevent cerebral edema. Blood pressure is recommended to control as systolic <180 mm Hg or mean arterial pressure <130 mm Hg, and lower blood pressure gradually to 80% of the baseline level. In case of acute cerebral infarction hypertension is not treated unless severely hypertensive, systolic >220 mm Hg or diastolic >120 mm Hg and lower blood pressure gradually to 85–90% of the baseline level. Use of warfarin is controversial in case of acute cerebral infarction. Modification of dialysis modality is needed to prevent the increase in intracranial pressure and/or recurrence of stroke.

Stroke Features in Dialysis Patients

In a previous publication [1], I wrote: 'Strokes, in particular cerebrovascular hemorrhage, were found to occur at a significantly higher rate in dialysis patients than in the general population. By logistic analysis, hypertension was demonstrated to be the single most reliable predictor of strokes; however, the risk was still elevated in dialysis patients with normal blood pressure. Therefore, the effects of uremia per se and malnutrition were thought to be the underlying causes of stroke. We suggest that strict blood pressure control, along with good nutritional support, should be effective in decreasing the incidence of stroke, particularly cerebral hemorrhages.' Since then the concept of chronic kidney disease (CKD) has been proposed and accepted widely [2, 3]. Currently, the dialysis patient is classified as CKD stage 5D. Early detection and early treatment of CKD is utmost important in both preventing progression to end-stage kidney disease (ESKD) and cardiovascular disease (CVD). CKD is a newly developed concept and has been accepted as a nonconventional (or kidney disease-related) risk factor of CVD and strokes (cerebrovascular disease, often included in CVD). Lower the kidney function (estimated glomerular filtration rate, GFR) and the number of risk factor increases. GFR is estimated simply by serum creatinine, age, and sex. Serum creatinine-based eGFR might be misleading among those with malnutrition and elderly population [4].

Criteria to start dialysis treatment depend on both eGFR and uremic symptoms. Since the uremic symptoms are not specific to CKD, initiation of dialysis therapy is often determined by low eGFR (<15 ml/min/1.73 m^2) only or empirically by the physician. 'Timely' start of dialysis is advisable; however, there are no criteria to start dialysis treatment using target eGFR and/or other intermediate markers. Dialysis therapy was expected to reduce the nonconventional risk factors in CKD stage 5 patients. Therefore, levels of eGFR at start of dialysis have been increased gradually in many countries, namely dialysis was started earlier than before. However, the higher the eGFR was at the start of dialysis, the worse was the prognosis [5, 6]. These observations suggested that hemodialysis per se might be harmful as it increased hemodynamic hazards such as sudden cardiac deaths and strokes. Otherwise, the findings were simply survival bias. Recent prospective randomized study showed that the survival rates were similar between those with early start (CCr 10–14 ml/min) and late start (CCr 5–7 ml/min) [7].

Epidemiology of Strokes

Incidence of cerebral hemorrhage is still high as 3.0–10.3 per 1,000 patient-years, which is more than 10 times higher than that of the general population [8]. Recently, the prevalence, and probably also the incidence of cerebral infarction, seemed to be increasing. This could be due to the changes in demographics of the incident dialysis patients. As shown, of the primary causes of ESKD by diabetes, hypertension is increasing whereas glomerulonephritis is decreasing (fig. 1) [9]. The prevalence of CVD was about 25% among the screened popula-

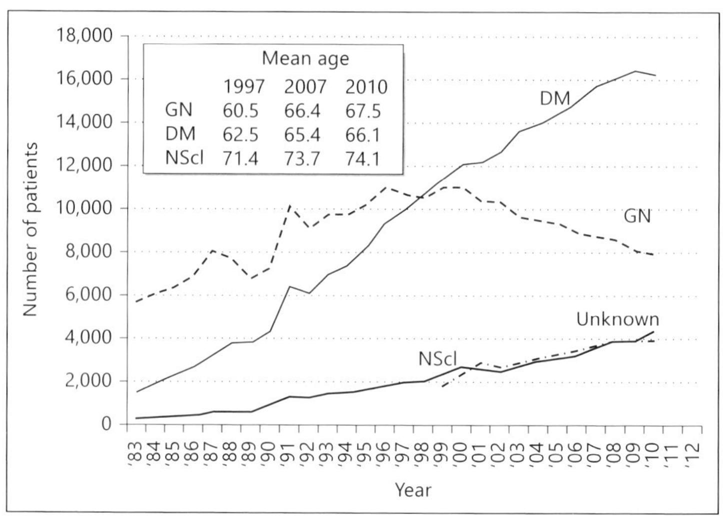

Fig. 1. Trends in primary kidney disease among Japanese incident dialysis patients [9].

tion at the level of CKD stage 4 in Japan [10]. Therefore, such high-risk patients, if they survived, would enter a dialysis program. The prognosis for hemodialysis patients with CVD is worse than that of the general population [11]. These findings support the concepts of CKD: the lower the eGFR, the higher the incidence of CVD and the death rate.

Pathophysiology

The mechanistic basis for the high incidence of stroke in dialysis patients is summarized in table 1. Dialysis patients have multiple risk factors and therefore they require many drugs. Compliance and adherence to their treatment strategy need to be monitored frequently. In this regard, an adequate dialysis regimen such as hemodialysis prescription of time and frequency and dialyzer (membrane and membrane area) is essential. Unfortunately, many intervention trials by erythropoietin-stimulating agents [12], dialysis dose [13] and statins [14] failed to show the treatment benefits including strokes. Dialysis-related complications increase in patients with larger interdialytic weight gain. Hemodynamic infarction which often occurs during and 6 h after a hemodialysis session [15] could be preventable if the interdialytic weight gain is controlled.

Diagnosis of CVD

In every dialysis patients, any neurological abnormality such as headache, paralysis, aphasia, dysarthria, anisocoria or convulsive attacks should be examined further to exclude CVD [8]. A precise diagnosis of stroke, location and nature

Table 1. Mechanistic basis for the high incidence of stroke in dialysis patients

1	Conventional risk factor	
	a	Hypertension
	b	Diabetes mellitus
	c	Dyslipidemia
	d	Smoking
	e	Aging
	f	Male
	g	White race
	h	Sedentary life style
	i	Menopause
	j	Left ventricular hypertrophy
	k	Sleep disorder (sleep apnea syndrome)
2	Nonconventional risk factor	
	a	Volume overload
	b	CKD-MBD (calcium, phosphate, parathyroid hormone)
	c	Anemia
	d	Oxidative stress (nitric oxide, endothelin)
	e	Sympathetic over-drive
	f	Malnutrition
	g	Dyslipidemia (triglyceride, lipoprotein)
	h	Homocystein
	i	Chronic inflammation (high CRP, low serum albumin)
	j	Sleep disturbance
3	Dialysis related factor	
	a	Hemodynamic
	b	Vascular access
	c	Dialysis amyloidosis
	d	Vascular calcification
	e	Dialysate (acetate)
	f	Dialysis vintage

using CT, MRI and MRI angiography should be made. Several radiographic tools are helpful, but the use of gadolinium is prohibited due to the occurrence of fibrosis of the nephrogenic systemic.

According to the annual registry data of the Japanese Society for Dialysis Therapy (JSDT), the prevalence of deaths due to stroke has been declining (fig. 2) [9]. Instead, deaths due to infection and malignancies are increasing. This trend may, at least partly, be reflecting the increased acceptance of patients with predialysis comorbid conditions such as CVD and malignancy. However, the role of changes in the incidence of CVD or the mortality rate after strokes is not clear. Stroke occurs frequently before and after starting dialysis treatment. Actually, the death hazard is higher within 6 months in incident dialysis patients.

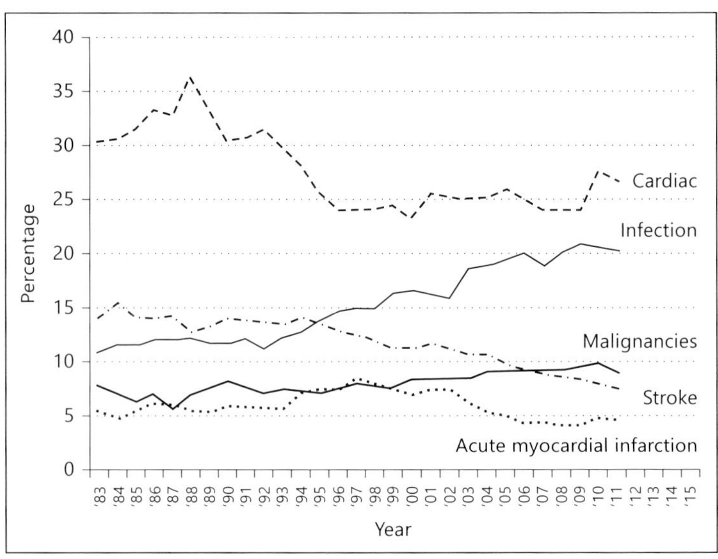

Fig. 2. Causes of death in prevalent dialysis patients [9].

Management

General and Dialysis Modality

In the case of cerebral hemorrhage, the larger the hematoma the poorer the prognosis. In the JSDT guideline, we recommend that hemodialysis should be avoided within 24 h after the onset (table 2) [8]. In the case of an acute indication of dialysis such as hyperkalemia, pulmonary edema, malignant hypertension, or uremic bleeding, medical treatment other than hemodialysis should be tried. Hemodialysis, if needed, should be performed with nafamostat mesilate as an anticoagulant. Glycerol should be used to prevent and treat cerebral edema. To prevent the recurrence or occurrence of stroke, the dose of hemodialysis should be minimized and, therefore, the amount of fluid and diet should be restricted for the first week after strokes. Vital signs should be monitored frequently.

Factors related to long-term survival of stroke patients are multifactorial, but maintaining a good nutritional status is of utmost important [16]. Causes of death among patients who survived the first month after the event are infection and malnutrition. Control of hyperphosphatemia is necessary to prevent vascular calcification and CKD-MBD. Coronary artery stenting and carotid endarterectomy are often performed in the nondialysis population, but so far they are of limited value among dialysis patients.

Table 2. Summary of care of stroke patients on dialysis: excerpt from the JSDT guidelines [8]

1 Cerebral bleeding
- a Control of brain edema: use glycerol with simultaneous ultrafiltration by dialysis. If needed, consult to neurosurgeon to remove hematoma or drainage. If the hematoma is too large, 30–50 ml, prognosis is very poor.
- b Control of blood pressure: maintain systolic (mean) blood pressure less than 180 (130) mm Hg.
- c Micro-bleeding. Dialysis patients may have higher prevalence.
- d Hematoma size: avoid hemodialysis within 24 h after the onset to prevent the increase in hematoma size. Some recommend initiating peritoneal dialysis.
- e Secondary prevention: To prevent the recurrence, it would be advisable to control blood pressure at around 140/90 mm Hg at pre-hemodialysis session.

2 Cerebral infarction
- a Blood pressure control: avoid aggressive control of blood pressure at acute phase. If blood pressure is very high (systolic >220 mm Hg, diastolic >120 mm Hg), start antihypertensive drugs. Target level is 85–90% of the baseline and lower blood pressure slowly.
- b Brain edema control: use glycerol with simultaneous fluid control by dialysis, but not on the day of event. Avoid acute hemodynamic change.
- c Anti-coagulation: use anti-platelet agents (aspirin, ticlopidine, clopidogrel, and cilostazol) or anticoagulants (argatroban, heparin, and warfarin). Need to consider the risk of bleeding. To prevent cerebral hemorrhage, periodical monitoring of PT-INR at <2.0 is recommended.
- d Primary prevention (atrial fibrillation): antithrombotic therapy, carotid endarterectomy, endovascular treatment, blood pressure control.
- e Secondary prevention (within 1 month): use antiplatelet, anticoagulant, or antihypertensives. Target level of blood pressure is 140/90 mm Hg, if patients have no evidence of bilateral carotid artery stenosis.

3. Subarachnoid hemorrhage
   Unfortunately, not enough studies are available to make any recommendations.

Blood Pressure

In the acute phase of cerebral hemorrhage, if blood pressure is as high as systolic blood pressure >180 mm Hg or mean blood pressure >130 mm Hg, use antihypertensive drugs gradually lowering the blood pressure until it reaches 80% of the previous value [8]. In the acute phase of cerebral infarction, no aggressive antihypertensive treatment is necessary unless it is associated with malignant hypertension. If hypertension is severe, e.g. systolic blood pressure >220 mm Hg or diastolic blood pressure >120 mm Hg, start antihypertensive treatment [8]. If the patient has indications for thrombolytic therapy, the target of antihypertensive treatment is <180/105 mm Hg, and antihypertensive drugs should be used to reduce the blood pressure until it reaches 85–90% of the previous value.

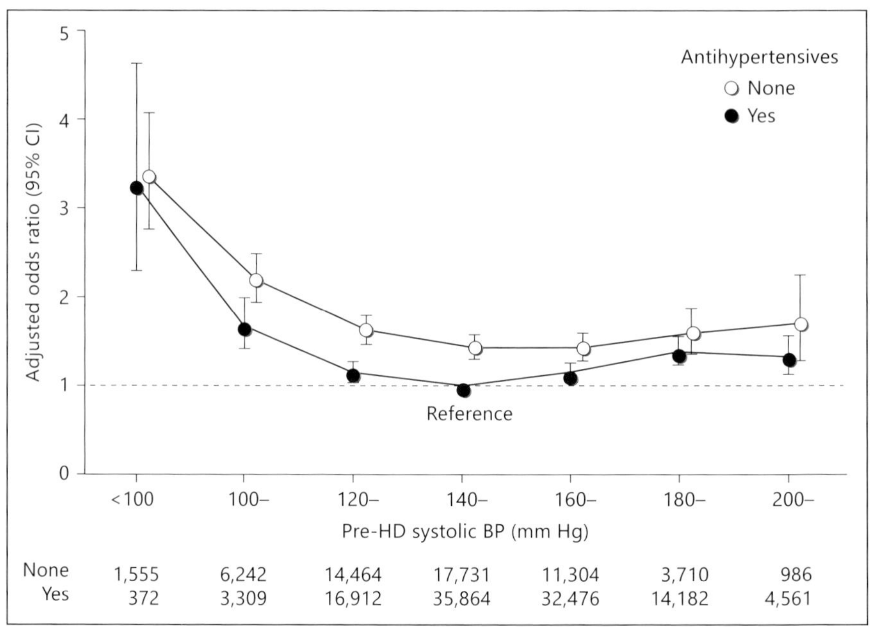

Fig. 3. Survival by systolic blood pressure taken before a hemodialysis session [19].

Secondary Prevention

Hypertension is a significant risk factor of stroke even in dialysis patients; however, the relationship between blood pressure level and survival is different from that of the nondialysis population [17, 18]. Prognosis is rather better in those with a high blood pressure of >140/90 mm Hg. We and others have shown better survival among those taking antihypertensive drugs regardless of the blood pressure levels (fig. 3) [19]. Several reports showed the benefit of angiotensin II receptor blockers (ARB) [20] or beta-blockers [21], but not of the combination of angiotensin-converting enzyme inhibitor (ACEI) plus ARB [22]. We have investigated the benefit of adding ARB (Olmesartan) for the treatment of hypertension, but there were no appreciable difference between ARB and non-ARB-based treatments on the primary event such as mortality rate, cardiac and CVD events [23].

Atrial Fibrillation

The prevalence of atrial fibrillation is higher among dialysis patients [8]. Contrary to the reports in a nondialysis population, the role of atrial fibrillation in the incidence of thrombotic infarction is not clear among dialysis patients. Warfarin has been used as an antithrombotic therapy and was effective for the secondary prevention of cardiogenic cerebral thrombosis in a nondialysis

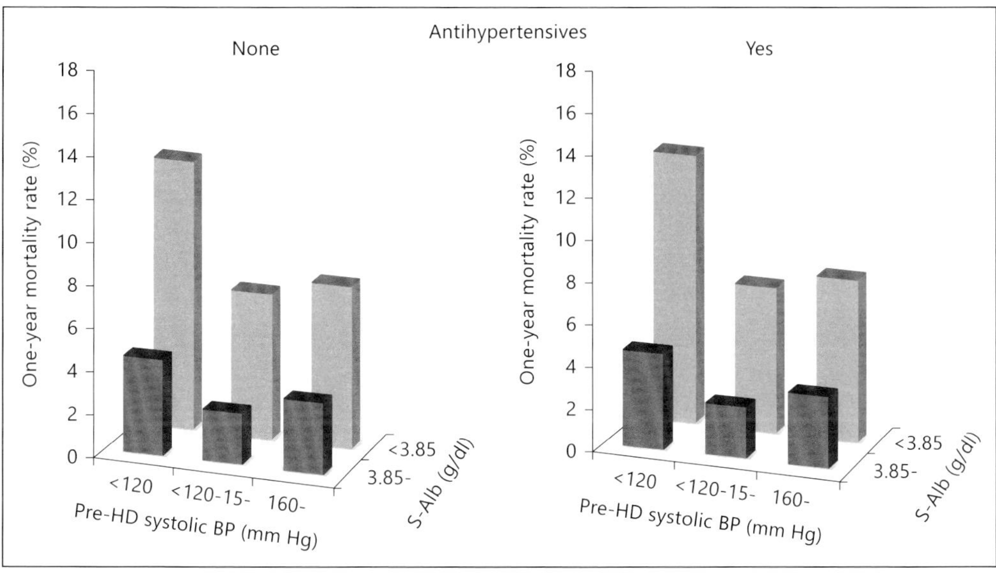

Fig. 4. Survival by blood pressure and serum albumin taken before a hemodialysis session [19].

population. Chan et al. [24] reported that the prognosis was poor in hemodialysis patients who were on anticoagulant agents such as warfarin, aspirin or clopidogrel, which probably increased the incidence of cerebral hemorrhage. Other than the anticoagulants, heparin which is commonly used in dialysis treatment and platelet dysfunction may increase the risk of cerebral hemorrhage, but not cerebral infarction. The INR (international normalized ratio) should be monitored regularly, if warfarin is indicated, and be maintained at INR <2.0 [25]. Dialysis patients often show tachycardia as the median was 74 per minute in the JSDT registry data [26]. The higher the pulse rate the poorer the prognosis, although the effect of atrial fibrillation per se was not determined in the study.

Malnutrition

The mortality rate of CVD is much higher in dialysis patients than that of the general population, in particular within 1 month of the event [27]. Dialysis patients are fragile and often contract infection. These complications are associated with malnutrition and chronic inflammation. Arteriovenous fistula and other vascular access are often failed in stroke patients. Therefore, they may become underdialyzed and suffer loss of appetite. Once hypoalbuminemia develops recovery is difficult. Other than monitoring calorie and protein intakes, adequate exercise should be encouraged. In this regard, a medical team of multiple staff should be organized [28]. Serum albumin is considered the intermediate marker of the well-being of the dialysis patients. According to the JSDT data, the prevalence of hypoalbuminemia (median value was 3.85 g/dl in the JSDT) was high and they were at a high risk of death (fig. 4) [29].

Future Problems

Stroke remains the major complication among the dialysis population. Regular dialysis treatment could not be continued as prescribed if the sequelae of stroke are severe, and the patient eventually develops malnutrition. Support for daily life and transportation to the dialysis unit often become difficult. Withdrawal from dialysis or reducing dialysis dose is becoming common practice [30]. For elderly patients with stroke, socioeconomic support is critical for the continuation of adequate dialysis.

References

1 Iseki K: Cerebrovascular Disease in ESRD; in Loscalzo J, London G (eds): The Cardiovascular Complications in End-Stage Renal Disease. Oxford, Oxford University Press, 2000, pp 443–461.

2 Matsushita K, van der Velde M, Astor BC, et al: Association of estimated glomerular filtration rate and albuminuria with all-cause and cardiovascular mortality in general population cohorts: a collaborative meta-analysis. Lancet 2010;375:2073–2081.

3 Levey A: Chronic kidney disease. Lancet 2012;379:165–180.

4 Matsuo S, Imai E, Horio M, et al: Revised equations for estimated GFR from serum creatinine in Japan. Am J Kidney Dis 2009;53: 982–992.

5 Wright S, Klausner D, Baird B, et al: Timing of dialysis initiation and survival in ESRD. Clin J Am Soc Nephrol 2010;5:1828–1835.

6 Rosansky SJ, Eggers P, Jackson K, et al: Early start of hemodialysis may be harmful. Arch Intern Med 2011;171:396–403.

7 Cooper BA, Branley P, Bulfone L, et al: A randomized, controlled trial of early versus late initiation of dialysis. N Engl J Med 2010; 363:600–619.

8 Hirakata H, Nitta K, Inaba M, et al: Japanese Society for Dialysis Therapy guidelines for management of cardiovascular diseases in patients on chronic hemodialysis. Ther Apheresis Dial 2012;16:387–435.

9 Nakai S, Iseki K, Itami N, et al: An overview of regular dialysis treatment in Japan (as of December 31, 2010). Ther Apheresis Dialysis 2012;16:483–521.

10 Iseki K, Asahi K, Moriyama T, et al: Risk factor profiles based on eGFR and dipstick proteinuria: analysis of the participants of the Specific Health Check and Guidance System in Japan 2008. Clin Exp Nephrol 2012;16: 244–249.

11 Iseki K, Wakugami K, Maehara A, et al: Long-term survival of chronic dialysis patients in comparison to that of stroke and acute myocardial infarction patients. Clin Exp Nephrol 2001;5:109–113.

12 Pfeffer MA, Burdmann EA, Chen CY, et al: A trial of darbepoetin alfa in type 2 diabetes and chronic kidney disease. N Engl J Med 2009; 361:2019–2032.

13 Eknoyan G, Beck GJ, Cheung AK, et al: Effect of dialysis dose and membrane flux in maintenance hemodialysis. N Engl J Med 2002; 347:2010–2019.

14 Wanner C, Krane V, Marz W, et al: Atorvastatin in patients with type 2 diabetes mellitus undergoing hemodialysis. N Engl J Med 2005;353:238–248.
15 Toyoda K, Fujii K, Fujimi S, et al: Stroke in patients on maintenance hemodialysis: a 22-year single-center study. Am J Kidney Dis 2005;45:1058–1066.
16 Iseki K, Shinzato T, Nagura Y, and Akiba T: Factors influencing long-term survival in patients on chronic dialysis. Clin Exp Nephrol 2004;8:89–97.
17 Iseki K: Reverse epidemiology in chronic hemodialysis patients. Nephrology Frontier 2007;6:82–83.
18 Kalantar-Zadeh K, Kilpatrick RD, McAllister CJ, et al: Reverse epidemiology of hypertension and cardiovascular death in the hemodialysis population. Hypertension 2005;45:811–817.
19 Iseki K, Shoji T, Nakai S, et al: Higher survival rates of chronic hemodialysis patients on antihypertensive drugs. Nephron Clin Pract 2009;113;C183–C190.
20 Takahashi A, Takase H, Toriyama T, et al: Candesartan, an angiotensin II type-1 receptor blocker, reduces cardiovascular events in patients on chronic haemodialysis – a randomized study. Nephrol Dial Transplant 2006;21:2507–2512.
21 Nakao K, Makino H, Morita S, et al: Beta-Blocker prescription and outcomes in hemodialysis patients from the Japan Dialysis Outcomes and Practice Patterns Study. Nephron Clin Pract 2009;113:132–139.
22 Chan KE, Ikizler TA, Gamboa JL, et al: K Combined angiotensin-converting enzyme inhibition and receptor blockade associate with increased risk of cardiovascular death in hemodialysis patients. Kidney Int 2011;80: 978–985.
23 Iseki K, Tokuyama K, Shiohira Y, et al: Olmesartan Clinical Trial in Okinawan Patients Under OKIDS Group (OCTOPUS): design and methods. Clin Exp Nephrol 2009; 13:145–151.
24 Chan KE, Lazarus JM, Thadhani R, Hakim RM: Anticoagulant and antiplatelet usage associates with mortality among hemodialysis patients. J Am Soc Nephrol 2009;20:872–881.
25 Chan KE, Lazarus JM, Thadhani R, Hakim RM: Warfarin use associates with increased risk for stroke in hemodialysis patients with atrial fibrillation. J Am Soc Nephrol 2009;20: 2223–2233.
26 Iseki K, Nakai S, Yamagata K, et al: Tachycardia as a predictor of poor survival in chronic hemodialysis patients. Nephrol Dial Transplant 2011;26:963–969.
27 Iseki K, Fukiyama K, and the Okinawa Dialysis Study (OKIDS) Group: Clinical demographics and long-term prognosis after stroke in patients on chronic hemodialysis. Nephrol Dial Transplant 2000;15:1808–1813.
28 Kalantar-Zadeh K, Burrowers JD, Franch H, et al: Nephrology and nutrition leaders coming to Hawaii for the World Renal Nutrition Week: Why is the 16th Congress in Renal Nutritional and Metabolism in Honolulu, Hawaii, June 2012, worth attending? J Ren Nutr 2012;22:1–3.
29 Iseki K, Shoji T, Nakai S, et al: Higher survival rates of chronic hemodialysis patients on antihypertensive drugs. Nephron Clin Pract 2009;113:C183–C190.
30 Germain MJ, Davison SN, Moss AH: When enough is enough: the nephrologist's responsibility in ordering dialysis treatment. Am J Kidney Dis 2001;58:135–143.

Kunitoshi Iseki, MD
Dialysis Unit, University Hospital of the Ryukyus
207 Uehara, Nishihara
Okinawa 903-0215 (Japan)
E-Mail chihokun@med.u-ryukyu.ac.jp

Toyoda K (ed): Brain, Stroke and Kidney.
Contrib Nephrol. Basel, Karger, 2013, vol 179, pp 110–118 (DOI: 10.1159/000346729)

Thrombolysis and Hyperacute Reperfusion Therapy for Stroke in Renal Patients

Teruyuki Hirano

Department of Neurology and Neuromuscular Disorders, Oita University Faculty of Medicine, Yufu, Japan

Abstract

Thrombolytic therapy using recombinant tissue plasminogen activator (rt-PA) is established as an effective treatment for patients with acute ischemic stroke. No distinction to the presence of chronic kidney disease (CKD) was made in previous clinical trials. In this chapter, three clinical studies that investigated renal dysfunction on the effect of rt-PA were reviewed and a meta-analysis was performed. In total, 344 patients with CKD and 504 patients without were treated within 3 h of symptom onset. Patients with CKD showed decreased odds of being alive and independent compared to patients with normal renal function (OR 0.60, 95% CI 0.45–0.81). Symptomatic intracranial hemorrhage occurred more in patients with CKD than without (OR 3.38, 95% CI 1.60–7.15). Risk of fatal outcome was also significantly higher in patients with CKD (OR 3.15, 95% CI 1.82–5.45).

Chronic Kidney Disease and Stroke

Chronic kidney disease (CKD) is identified as a risk factor for stroke in the general population [1, 2], as well as in high-risk patients having diabetes mellitus [3], essential hypertension [4], and preexisting atherothrombotic disease [5]. In a large cohort of patients with acute stroke, CKD was an independent predictor for long-term mortality and poor outcome [6, 7]. Patients with CKD are known to have abnormalities in coagulation and platelet function that favor thrombosis in the untreated state and the augment bleeding risks in the setting of antiplatelet drugs and anticoagulants. Prior studies have demonstrated that increased levels of thrombin generation, circulating thrombin-antithrombin complex and plasminogen activator inhibitor. The systemic atherosclerotic vascular disease process seen with CKD may partly explain its association with stroke [8]. Cardiovascular risk factors including hypertension, insulin resistance, endothelial dysfunction and inflammation are highly prevalent. Small-vessel cerebrovascular disease has also been described in CKD patients.

Mechanism of Stroke

Vascular occlusion in the cerebral circulation results in ischemic of cerebral tissue that causes tissue infarction. Approximately 80% of strokes are ischemic. Main pathophysiologic mechanisms of stroke are thrombosis, embolism, or altered coagulation. In general, renal patients suffer from stroke with thromboembolism as a result of atherosclerosis, inflammation, and cardioembolism.

Large- and Medium-Sized Artery Stenosis

In the large- and medium-sized arteries of the brain or neck, atherosclerosis leads to either thrombotic vessel occlusion or artery-to-artery embolism. The distribution of atherosclerotic plaques varies by gender and race [9, 10]. The accelerated progression of atherosclerosis in this population, which may begin during advanced chronic renal dysfunction, can be related to a number of factors that are unique to advanced kidney disease, namely elevated calcium-phosphate product, hyperhomocysteinemia, inflammation, oxidative stress and anemia [11].

Lacunar Strokes

Lacunes are defined as small (<15 mm in diameter), deep cerebral infarcts. They are common, causing approximately 20% of all ischemic strokes. These infarcts are most often found in the white matter, basal ganglia, thalamus, pons, and cerebellum. Since the earliest descriptions, lacunar stroke has been considered to be due to pathology of the small penetrating arteries of the brain [12], whereas large- and medium-sized arteries are affected by atherosclerosis. It is unclear whether this process also affects the microscopic penetrating arteries of the brain that lead to these small lacunar infarcts [12]. Hypertension was thought to be the main cause of disease of the penetrating artery of the brain and, therefore, the cause of lacunar infarcts, but hypertension has been shown to be no more important in the development of lacunes compared with other types of stroke [13].

The paucity of autopsy material in patients with lacunar stroke has made it difficult to define a particular arteriopathy in these clinically defined syndromes [13].

Emboli

Emboli can arise from the heart, aorta, carotids, or vertebrobasilar system. Cardiac disorders that give rise to embolism can be grouped into six categories: (1) arrhythmias; (2) valvular heart disease; (3) ventricular myocardial structural abnormalities, such as aneurysms, dilated cardiomyopathies, and akinetic walls; (4) intraventricular masses, myxoma, or other tumors; (5) shunts, especially intra-atrial septal defects (patent foramen ovale alone is no longer considered a risk factor for stroke, but it is a risk factor if there is an associated atrial septal aneurysms), and (6) atrial lesions, such as dilated atria, thrombi, tumors and infarcts.

Thrombolysis for Acute Ischemic Stroke

Thrombolytic therapy with intravenous (i.v.) recombinant tissue plasminogen activator (rt-PA) was established as an effective treatment of acute ischemic stroke in patients presenting within 3 h of symptom onset, according to the results of the National Institutes of Neurological Disorders and Stroke (NINDS) rt-PA trial published in 1995 [14]. This therapy was effective regardless of the type of ischemic stroke. In 2008, the 3-hour time window was extended to 4.5 h, when the third European Cooperative Acute Stroke Trial (ECASS3) showed significant increase of a favorable outcome (modified Rankin scale (mRS) 0–1, OR 1.34, 95% CI 1.02–1.76) [15] in patients treated between 3 and 4.5 h after the symptom onset. The systematic review of i.v. rt-PA updated in 2012, including the results of the third international stroke trial (IST-3) [16], indicated that rt-PA given within 6 h of stroke significantly increased the odds of being alive and independent (mRS 0–2) at 6 months (OR 1.17, 95% CI 1.06–1.29), absolute increase of 42 (95% CI 19–66) per 1,000 people treated [17]. The benefit of rt-PA was greatest in patients treated within 3 h (mRS 0–2, OR 1.53, 1.26–1.86), absolute benefit of 90 (46–135) per 1,000 people treated.

The major complication of i.v. rt-PA is symptomatic intracranial hemorrhage (ICH) causing increased disability or death. In fact, numbers of deaths within 7 days were increased (OR 1.44, 95% CI 1.18–1.76), and symptomatic ICH accounted for most of the early excess deaths (OR 3.72, 95% CI 2.98–4.64) on the systematic review [17].

Table 1. Studies evaluating the effect of i.v. rt-PA in patients with vs. without CKD

	Lyrer et al. [18] (2008) (n = 196)		Agrawal et al. [19] (2010) (n = 74)		Naganuma et al. [20] (2011), (n = 578)	
Definition of CKD	GFR <90		eGFR <60		eGFR <60	
Number of CKD patients	138		20		186	
Dosage of alteplase, mg/kg	0.9		0.9		0.6	
Outcome assessment	3 months		at discharge		3 months	
	%	p	%	p	%	p
mRS						
0–1			15.0 vs. 31.5	0.156	25.8 vs. 38.0	0.004
0–2	53.6 vs. 70.7	0.038				
3–6			70.0 vs. 57.4	0.324		
4–6					47.9 vs. 34.7	0.003
Death	15.9 vs. 6.9	–	10.0 vs. 7.4	0.717	13.4 vs. 3.8	<0.001
Any ICH			20.0 vs. 11.1	0.321		
Symptomatic ICH	8.0 vs. 1.7	0.038	0 vs. 1.9	n.s.	8.1 vs. 2.6	0.004

Effect of Intravenous rt-PA in Stroke Patients with CKD

Many clinical trials have demonstrated improved neurological outcomes with i.v. rt-PA therapy but with an increased risk for ICH as a potential serious complication [14, 15, 17]. Because no distinction to the presence of CKD was made in established randomized-controlled clinical trials, major guidelines are silent on this issue. One comment in the guideline warns that 'any other condition that could increase the risk of hemorrhage after alteplase administration' is a reason for withholding treatment with i.v. rt-PA.

To date, 3 studies have assessed whether CKD influences outcomes in patients treated with i.v. rt-PA for acute ischemic stroke [18–20] (table 1). In these studies, the presence of CKD was determined by impaired estimated glomerular filtration rate (eGFR). Definition of CKD in each study was eGFR <60 in two [19, 20] and the remaining employed <90 ml/min/1.73 m^2 [18]. Alteplase was used in all, but the dosage (0.9 or 0.6 mg/kg) was different according to the guideline of the particular countries. Two studies assessed the mRS at 3 months [18, 20]; however, one retrospective study used outcome assessment of hospital discharge [19]. In summary, the two larger studies [18, 20] reported CKD to be associated with higher rates of symptomatic ICH after rt-PA treatment; this association was independent of other recognized risk factors in the Japanese Stroke Acute Management with Urgent Risk-Factor Assessment and Improvement (SAMURAI) rt-PA registry [20]. One study also demonstrated impaired renal function before thrombolysis is associated with increased odds for a poor outcome [18].

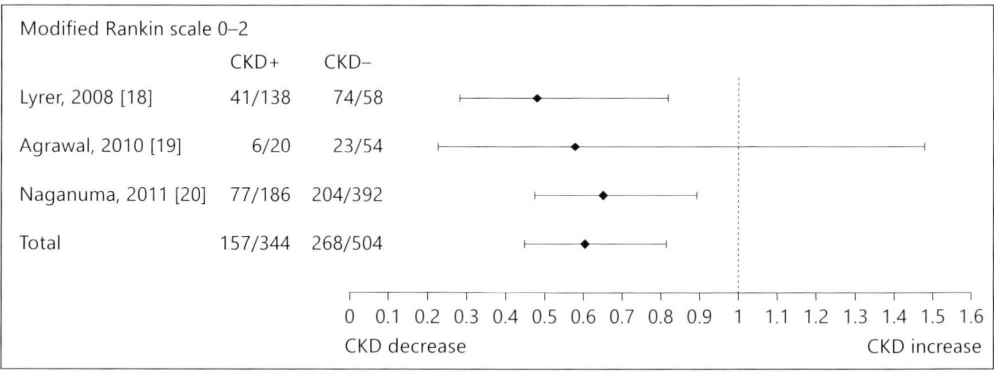

Fig. 1. Effect of CKD on alive and independent stroke patients with rt-PA therapy. Data are numbers (OR 0.60, 95% CI 0.45–0.81), Mantel-Haenszel methods.

Efficacy of i.v. rt-PA in Terms of Clinical Outcome

After reaching a consensus of the differences in study designs, a meta-analysis was performed to clarify the effect of i.v. rt-PA in stroke patients with CKD. In total, 344 patients with CKD and 504 patients without CKD were treated within 3 h of symptom onset. Patients with CKD had significantly decreased odds of being alive and independent (mRS 0–2) compared to patients with normal renal function (157/344 [45.6%] vs. 268/504 [53.2%], OR 0.60, 95% CI 0.45–0.81) (fig. 1).

Renal dysfunction is associated with traditional vascular risk factors, including aging, hypertension, diabetes mellitus, dyslipidemia, and smoking. In addition, CKD is now known to be an independent predictor of stroke [21], partly via nontraditional vascular risk factors, e.g. inflammatory factors, and homocysteinemia. Moreover, renal dysfunction might impair endothelial release of t-PA [22], and increase plasminogen activator inhibitor-1 activity [23] and plasma levels of lipoprotein(a). These abnormalities might obstruct the reperfusion phenomenon and worsen stroke outcome after i.v. rt-PA.

Symptomatic ICH

Definition of symptomatic ICH was in accord with the NINDS rt-PA study definition, such as any ICH defined as CT or MRI evidence of new ICH with neurological deterioration corresponding to an increase of ≥1 point from the baseline NIHSS score. Presence of CKD was significantly related to symptomatic ICH (26/344 [7.6%] vs. 12/504 [2.4%], OR 3.38, 95% CI 1.60–7.15) (fig. 2).

It can be hypothesized that chronic microvascular damage to the cerebral blood vessels in CKD may predispose these vessels to further injury and rupture in the setting of an acute stroke after thrombolytic therapy. A hemorrhagic

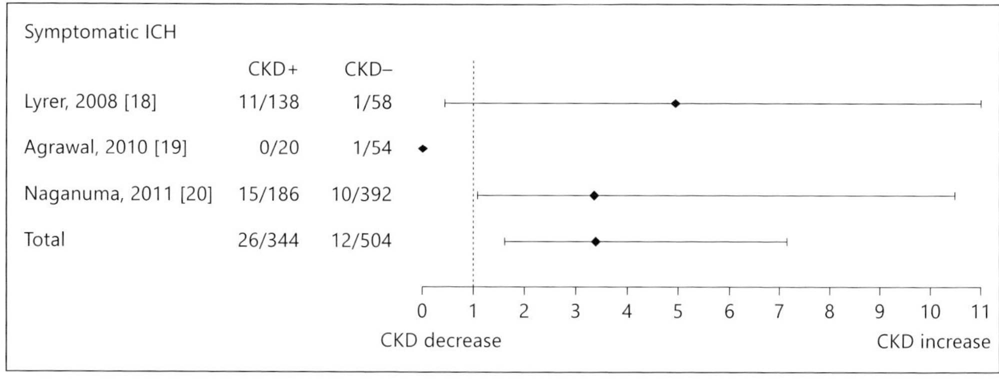

Fig. 2. Effect of CKD on symptomatic ICH after rt-PA therapy. Data are numbers (OR 3.38, 95% CI 1.60–7.15), Mantel-Haenszel methods.

transformation of the infarct may thus be possible from reperfusion injury when rt-PA recanalize the occluded blood vessels. Abnormalities in platelet function and platelet-endothelial interactions in CKD may increase the bleeding risk in these patients. These disturbances may offset the beneficial effect of rt-PA in CKD as suggested by a clinical trial of rt-PA use in acute myocardial infarction [24].

Death after Thrombolysis

During the 3-month follow-up period, 72/848 (8.5%) patients died. In patients with CKD, causes of death were malignant brain infarction (15/47 [31.9%]), pneumonia (9/47 [19.1%]), myocardial infarction/pulmonary embolism (4/47 [8.5%]), heart failure (4/47 [8.5%]), sepsis (3/47 [6.3%]), infectious endocarditis (1/47 [2.1%]), symptomatic ICH (1/47 [2.1%]), and unknown (10/47 [21.3%]). On the other hand, patients without CKD died from malignant brain infarction (12/19 [63.2%]), pneumonia (2/19 [10.5%]) and unknown (5/19 [26.3%]) [18, 20]. Risk of fatal outcome was significantly higher in patients with CKD (49/344 [14.2%] vs. 23/504 [4.6%], OR 3.15, 95% CI 1.82–5.45) (fig. 3).

Neuroendovascular Reperfusion Therapies

The possibility that administration of thrombolytic agent into clot directly might lead to more rapid or efficient recanalization and allow for treatment further from symptom onset has led to studies of catheter-based intra-arterial thrombolysis. A meta-analysis of major catheter-based thrombolysis including PRO-

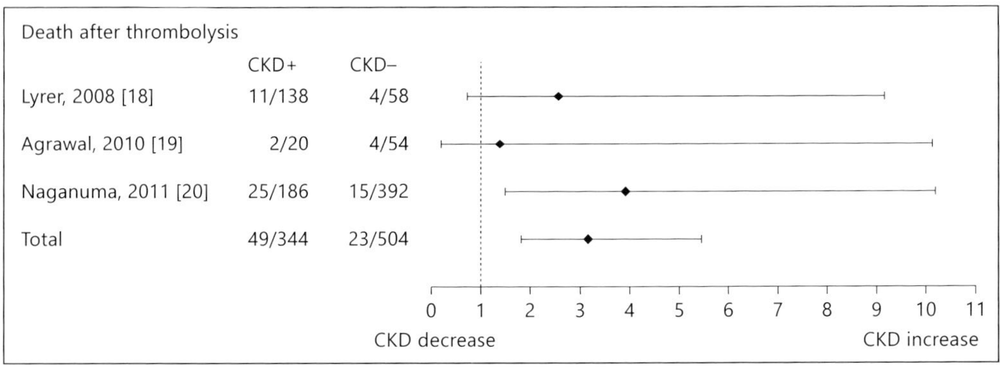

Fig. 3. Effect of CKD on fatal outcome after rt-PA therapy. Data are numbers (OR 3.15, 95% CI 1.82–5.45), Mantel-Haenszel methods.

ACT2 (Prolyse in Acute Cerebral Thromboembolism) [25] and MELT (Middle Cerebral Artery Embolism Local Fibrinolytic Intervention Trial) Japan [26] showed significantly reduced rate of death or dependency (OR 0.58, 95% CI 0.36–0.93) in patients treated within 6 hours of onset using catheter-delivered prourokinase or urokinase [27]. Although not statistically significant, more symptomatic ICH was observed in both studies (PROACT2, 10 vs. 2%; MELT, 9 vs. 2%).

Mechanical thrombectomy is another approach to achieve acute reperfusion. Rapid and dramatic development of new-generation devices, such as Merci [28], Penumbra [29] and Solitaire [30] could reduce amount or avoid use of thrombolytics and resulting in lower complication rate of ICH. However, use of contrast agent remained as inevitable negative factor for neuroendovascular therapies.

References

1 Yuyun MF, Khaw KT, Luben R, et al: Microalbuminuria and stroke in a British population: the European Prospective Investigation into Cancer in Norfolk (EPIC-Norfolk) population study. J Intern Med 2004;255:247–256.

2 Ninomiya T, Kiyohara Y, Kubo M, et al: Chronic kidney disease and cardiovascular disease in a general Japanese population: the Hisayama Study. Kidney Int 2005;68:228–236.

3 Guerrero-Romero F, Rodríguez-Morán M: Proteinuria is an independent risk factor for ischemic stroke in non-insulin-dependent diabetes mellitus. Stroke 1999;30:1787–1791.

4 De Leeuw PW, This L, Birkenhäger WH, et al: Prognostic significance of renal function in elderly patients with isolated systolic hypertension: results from the Syst-Eur Trial. J Am Soc Nephrol 2002;13:2213–2222.

5 Klausen KP, Scharling H, Jensen JS: Very low level of microalbuminuria is associated with increased risk of death in subjects with cardiovascular or cerebrovascular diseases. J Intern Med 2006;260:231–237.
6 Yahalom G, Schwartz R, Schwammenthal Y, et al: Chronic kidney disease and clinical outcome in patients with acute stroke. Stroke 2009;40:1296–1303.
7 Tsagalis G, Akrivos T, Alevizaki M, et al: Renal dysfunction in acute stroke: an independent predictor of long-term all combined vascular events and overall mortality. Nephrol Dial Transplant 2009;24:194–200.
8 Shoji T, Emoto M, Tabata T, et al. Advanced atherosclerosis in predialysis patients with chronic renal failure. Kidney Int 2002;61: 2187–2192.
9 Seliger SL, Gillen DL, Longstreth WT Jr, et al: Elevated risk of stroke among patients with end-stage renal disease. Kidney Int 2003;64: 603–609.
10 Toyoda K, Fujii K, Kumai Y, et al: Stroke in patients on maintenance hemodialysis: a 22-year single-center study. Am J Kidney Dis. 2005;45:1058–1066.
11 Abramson JL, Jurkovitz CT, Vaccarino V, et al: Chronic kidney disease, anemia, and incident stroke in a middle-aged, community-based population: The ARIC Study. Kidney Int 2003;64:610–615.
12 Mohr JP: Lacunar stroke. Hypertension 1986; 8:349–356.
13 Lodder J, Bamford JM, Sandercock PA, et al: Are hypertension or cardiac embolism likely causes of lacunar infarction? Stroke 1990;21: 375–381.
14 The National Institute of Neurological Disorders and Stroke rt-PA Stroke Study Group: Tissue plasminogen activator for acute ischemic stroke. N Engl J Med 1995;333:1581–1587.
15 Hacke W, Kaste M, Bluhmki E, et al: Thrombolysis with alteplase 3–4.5 h after acute ischemic stroke. N Engl J Med 2008;359:1317–1329.
16 The IST-3 collaborative group: The benefits and harms of intravenous thrombolysis with recombinant tissue plasminogen activator within 6 h of acute ischaemic stroke (the third international stroke trial [IST-3]): a randomised controlled trial. Lancet 2012;379: 2352–2363.
17 Wardlaw JM, Murray V, Berge E, et al: Recombinant tissue plasminogen activator for acute ischaemic stroke: an updated systematic review and meta-analysis. Lancet 2012; 379:2364–2372.
18 Lyrer PA, Fluri F, Gisler D, et al: Renal function and outcome among stroke patients treated with IV thrombolysis. Neurology 2008;71:1548–1550.
19 Agrawal V, Rai B, Fellows J, et al: In-hospital outcomes with thrombolytic therapy in patients with renal dysfunction presenting with acute ischaemic stroke. Nephrol Dial Transplant 2010;25:1150–1157.
20 Naganuma M, Koga M, Shiokawa Y, et al: Reduced estimated glomerular filtration rate is associated with stroke outcome after intravenous rt-PA: the Stroke Acute Management with Urgent Risk-Factor Assessment and Improvement (SAMURAI) rt-PA Registry. Cerebrovasc Dis 2011;31:123–129.
21 Go AS, Chertow GM, Fan D, et al: Chronic kidney disease and the risks of death, cardiovascular events, and hospitalization. N Engl J Med 2004;351:1296–1305.
22 Hrafnkelsdóttir T, Ottosson P, Gudnason T, et al: Impaired endothelial release of tissue-type plasminogen activator in patients with chronic kidney disease and hypertension. Hypertension 2004;44:300–304.
23 Kamgar M, Nobakhthaghighi N, Shamshirsaz AA, et al: Impaired fibrinolytic activity in type II diabetes: correlation with urinary albumin excretion and progression of renal disease Kidney Int 2006;69:1899–1903.
24 Gibson CM, Pinto DS, Murphy SA, et al: Association of creatinine and creatinine clearance on presentation in acute myocardial infarction with subsequent mortality. J Am Coll Cardiol 2003;42:1535–1543.
25 Furlan A, Higashida R, Wechsler L, et al: Intra-arterial prourokinase for acute ischemic stroke. The PROACT II study: a randomized controlled trial. JAMA 1999;282:2003–2011.
26 Ogawa A, Mori E, Minematsu K, et al: Randomized trial of intraarterial infusion of urokinase within 6 hours of middle cerebral artery stroke: the Middle Cerebral Artery Embolism Local Fibrinolytic Intervention Trial (MELT) Japan. Stroke 2007;38:2633–2639.

27 Saver JL: Intra-arterial fibrinolysis for acute ischemic stroke: the message of Melt. Stroke 2007;38:2627–2628.
28 Smith WS, Sung G, Saver J: Mechanical thrombectomy for acute ischemic stroke: final results of the Multi MERCI trial. Stroke 2008;39:1205–1212.
29 The Penumbra Pivotal Stroke Trial Investigators: Safety and effectiveness of a new generation of mechanical devices for clot removal in intracranial large vessel occlusive disease. Stroke 2009;40:2761–2768.
30 Castaño C, Dorado L, Guerrero C, et al: Mechanical thrombectomy with the Solitaire AB device in large artery occlusions of the anterior circulation: υ pilot study. Stroke 2010;41:1826–1840.

Teruyukı Hirano, MD, PhD
Department of Neurology and Neuromuscular Disorders
Oita University Faculty of Medicine
1-1 Idaigaoka, Hasama, Yufu, 879-5593 (Japan)
E-Mail terry12@oita-u.ac.jp

Toyoda K (ed): Brain, Stroke and Kidney.
Contrib Nephrol. Basel, Karger, 2013, vol 179, pp 119–129 (DOI: 10.1159/000346730)

Antiplatelet Therapy for Preventing Stroke in Patients with Chronic Kidney Disease

Suk Jae Kim · Oh Young Bang

Department of Neurology, Samsung Medical Center, Sungkyunkwan University School of Medicine, Seoul, Korea

Abstract

Chronic kidney disease (CKD), defined as reduced glomerular filtration rate and/or proteinuria, is a serious worldwide health problem. The incidence and prevalence of CKD are increasing with age, and patients with CKD are a population at very high risk for developing stroke. CKD may increase the risk for incident stroke independent of conventional stroke risk factors. A common pathological process including anemia, homocysteine, nitric oxide, oxidative stress, inflammation, and conditions promoting coagulation may be related to the development of stroke in the course of CKD. CKD can also serve as a marker of brain injury, because the cerebral microvascular system has similar hemodynamic features with the vascular beds of the kidney. CKD has been linked with markers of cerebral small artery disease including white matter lesions, lacunar infarctions, and cerebral microbleeds. CKD has been implicated with neurological deterioration during hospitalization, poor functional outcome, and hemorrhagic transformation in patients with acute stroke. Recurrence of stroke may also be higher in CKD patients compared with those having normal kidney function. However, there have been no specific recommendations for antiplatelet therapy in patients with ischemic stroke plus CKD. As CKD patients have distinct characteristics including high bleeding complications and poor response to antiplatelet agents, selecting and adjusting platelet aggregation inhibitors should be individualized. In addition, it should be noted that aspirin may aggravate renal dysfunction. Phosphodiesterase inhibitors restore endothelial dysfunction and may serve as a target for preventing stroke in CKD patients. Aside from antiplatelet therapy, other treatments including lipid control, blood pressure lowering, and renal transplantation are also important. Further studies are warranted for optimal treatment in stroke prevention in CKD patients.

Chronic kidney disease (CKD), defined as reduced glomerular filtration rate (GFR) and/or proteinuria, is a serious condition and a worldwide public health problem [1]. The incidence and prevalence of CKD are increasing with age, and it is associated with poor outcomes and a high cost to the healthcare system. Herein, we describe the relationship between brain and kidney, characteristics of stroke in patients with CKD, antiplatelet therapy for patients with ischemic stroke plus CKD, and various treatment strategies other than antiplatelet agents for prevention of stroke in CKD patients.

Brain and Kidney

CKD as a Risk Factor for Stroke

Since many traditional stroke risk factors also serve as risk factors for CKD, including older age, hypertension, diabetes mellitus (DM), and smoking, it appears clear that individuals with CKD are a population at very high risk for developing stroke. However, it is controversial whether CKD itself independently causes incident stroke [1]. Although CKD is an independent risk factor for cardiovascular disease (CVD) events among the general population [2], there have been inconsistent data regarding the link between CKD and incident stroke.

Recently, some studies have found that CKD may increase a risk for stroke events independently of conventional risk factors [3, 4]. A common pathological process including anemia, homocysteine, nitric oxide, oxidative stress, inflammation, and conditions promoting coagulation may be related to the development of stroke in the course of CKD [3]. On the other hand, one population-based study revealed that CKD is a stroke risk factor for only hemorrhagic stroke [5]. A recent study that found that CKD is associated with enhanced risk of hemorrhagic stroke for men and of ischemic stroke for women suggests that the relationship between CKD and risk of stroke and its subtype may be sex-specific [6].

CKD as a Marker of Brain Injury

The cerebral microvascular system has similar hemodynamic features with the vascular beds of the kidney, along with the retina. Kidney dysfunction is associated with endothelial dysfunction and lipohyalinosis [7], both of which are also hallmarks of small vessel disease (SAD) in the brain. Therefore, CKD may serve as a marker of brain injury. In this context, there has been considerable interest devoted to the relationship between kidney function and cerebral SAD.

The Northern Manhattan community-based cohort study clearly showed the association of CKD with white matter hyperintensity volume [8]. Similarly, another population-based investigation, the Rotterdam Scan Study, revealed the link between kidney dysfunction and markers of cerebral SAD including white matter lesions and lacunar infarcts [9]. A recent retrospective analysis found that impaired renal function was also related to cerebral microbleeds, which are another indicator of cerebral SAD in acute ischemic stroke [10]. Although the exact mechanisms are unclear, it has been speculated that CKD leads to brain injury directly or indirectly by mitigating the effects of stroke risk factors including hypertension and diabetes, rather than simply shared damages [11].

Characteristics of Stroke in CKD Patients

Clinical Outcome after Stroke in CKD Patients

The association between CKD and increased cardiovascular morbidity and mortality compared with the general population has been established [12]. The prevalence of CKD increases with age, as it does for stroke incidence, raising the possibility that CKD can be a predictor of clinical outcome after stroke. Some studies have found that low estimated GFR (eGFR) can be a strong predictor of mortality after stroke, especially short-term one [13]. On the other hand, one recent study demonstrated that low eGFR is a distinct long-term predictor of mortality after ischemic stroke only in patients younger than 65-years of age [14]. Low eGFR or the presence of CKD is also associated with neurological deterioration during hospitalization, poor functional outcome, and hemorrhagic transformation in patients with acute stroke [15, 16].

Recurrent Stroke in CKD Patients

There is a paucity of data regarding stroke recurrence in patients with CKD. Previous studies of patients with unstable coronary syndromes found that the presence of CKD is associated with subsequent CVD [17]. Similarly, a study of 4,278 subjects with pre-existing CVD from four community-based, longitudinal studies revealed that those with CKD had a 1.35-fold hazard ratio of recurrent cardiovascular events compared with those with normal kidney function [18]. Subgroup analysis also revealed that a significantly greater percentage of subjects with CKD experienced recurrent stroke with a 1.30-fold hazard ratio [18]. Recently, one observational study reported that CKD exhibited a 1.73-fold hazard ratio of recurrent non-cardioembolic stroke [19]. These findings may suggest that preventing deterioration in CKD could be an efficacious target for the prevention of stroke recurrence.

Antiplatelet Therapy for Preventing Stroke in CKD Patients

Current Guidelines for Antiplatelet Therapy in Non-Cardioembolic Stroke Patients

There have been several guidelines for antiplatelet therapy for secondary prevention of non-cardioembolic ischemic stroke [20, 21]. All guidelines recommend aspirin, combined aspirin and dipyridamole (Aggrenox®), or clopidogrel as an initial choice of therapy. A recent guideline also suggests cilostazol or triflusal as an alternative, especially for patients with a high-risk of bleeding [22]. However, there have been no specific recommendations for antiplatelet therapy in patients with ischemic stroke plus CKD.

Considerations in Selecting Antiplatelet Agents for CKD Patients

As patients with CKD have a higher risk of stroke and poor outcome after stroke than those without CKD, the treatment for prevention of stroke is quite important in this group of patients. Antiplatelet therapy is a mainstay of prevention of noncardioembolic ischemic stroke. Selection and adjusting antiplatelet agents should be individualized on the basis of patient's risk factors, stroke subtypes, and renal conditions.

Hemorrhage Risk

Patients with advanced kidney disease are prone to hemorrhage when treated with antiplatelet agents. Bleeding complications occur in these patients despite a normal coagulation profile or elevated coagulation factors, suggesting that abnormal platelet function may be related to hemorrhagic events [23]. The platelet response to vessel injury including platelet activation, recruitment, adhesion, and aggregation is defective, due to both intrinsic platelet abnormalities and impaired platelet-vessel wall interaction in advanced kidney disease [24].

A post hoc subgroup analysis of a randomized controlled trial revealed that among every 1,000 persons with eGFR <45 ml/min/1.73 m^2 treated with aspirin for 3.8 years, 27 excess major bleeds occurred, although the increased risk of the complication appeared to be outweighed by the profound benefits [25]. Conversely, a meta-analysis showed that there was no significant difference of major extracranial bleeds between antiplatelet and adjusted control groups [27/1,333 (2.0%) antiplatelet vs. 31/1,371 (2.3%) control], while the benefits of antiplatelet therapy in patients with CKD were consistent [26]. The risk-benefit analysis of antiplatelet therapy can possibly be applied to the CKD plus stroke patients, but exact figures are not available.

Increased Platelet Agglutinability and Resistance to Antiplatelet Agents

The responsiveness to antiplatelet agents including aspirin and clopidogrel differs considerably among individual subjects. Platelet responsiveness to antiplatelet drugs is lower in patients with CKD than in those with normal kidney function [27]. As opposed to enhanced bleeding complications, a prothrombotic state is also present in patients with CKD. It is characterized by increases in fibrinogen, von Willebrand factor, and tissue factor and a decrease in antithrombin III [28]. In addition, an increase in the platelet turnover rate and poor bioabilities including decreased absorption or drug transportation could contribute to increased thrombogenic potential in CKD [27, 29].

It has been reportedly found that 5–45% of patients receiving aspirin and 4–30% of those taking clopidogrel showed resistance to the antiplatelet drugs. The platelet responsiveness to P2Y12 receptor-mediated drugs such as clopidogrel is reduced more in patients with type 2 DM than in nondiabetic patients and type 2 DM is a key risk factor for CKD. Therefore, one may assume that poor antiplatelet responsiveness in CKD occurs because of an underlying cause of CKD, such as DM. However, the decreased platelet inhibition was improved by an increase in the clopidogrel dose in patients with DM, but not in those with CKD [27]. Moreover, one recent study conducted among patients with DM and coronary artery disease taking maintenance aspirin and clopidogrel therapy found that CKD itself was associated with reduced clopidogrel-induced antiplatelet effects [30].

Considering the low response to antiplatelet agents in CKD, additional investigations addressing the overcoming of antiplatelet resistance is essential in these high-risk patients. A recent study reported that adding cilostazol to clopidogrel (75 mg) improves platelet inhibition compared with 75–150 mg of clopidogrel alone in CKD patients undergoing hemodialysis and percutaneous coronary intervention [31]. Data from stroke plus CKD patients regarding antiplatelet responsiveness are currently lacking, and future studies in this subject are warranted.

Endothelial Dysfunction

Since endothelial dysfunction may be a link between CKD and ischemic stroke, it is conceivable that strategies to restore endothelial dysfunction may be important in preventing stroke in CKD patients. Various strategies are reported to reverse endothelial dysfunction. These include lifestyle modification (exercise, smoking cessation), risk factors control using statins or angiotensin converting enzyme inhibitors, L-arginine supplementation, and tetrahydrobiopterin to augment nitric oxide and anti-oxidants production.

Evidence is mounting that phosphodiesterase inhibitors (such as cilostazol and dipyridamole) increase nitric oxide and restore endothelial dysfunction. Recent large randomized trials showed that, compared to aspirin, cilostazol significantly reduced stroke recurrence especially SAD (a major stroke subtype in CKD patients) with a reduced risk of bleeding [32]. Further studies are needed evaluating the effects of strategies targeting on endothelial dysfunction in patients with CKD.

Effects of Antiplatelet Therapy on Renal Impairment

Aside from the increased risk of hemorrhage in CKD patients treated with aspirin, the use of aspirin has been debated due to the suspicion that aspirin increases the risk of renal impairment [33]. A previous study documented that regular use of aspirin was associated with an increased risk of chronic renal failure by a factor of 2.5 compared with that for non-users; the relative risk rose with increasing cumulative lifetime doses of aspirin and with increasing average doses during periods of regular use, but not with an increasing duration of use of aspirin [34]. Although the study could not rule out the possibility of bias owing to triggering of analgesic consumption by predisposing conditions, the findings suggested that great caution is needed when antiplatelet agents are administered in patients with CKD.

On the other hand, there has been no clear evidence of cilostazol-related renal impairment, even though it is recommended to use cilostazol with caution in patients with severe renal impairment. In addition, several pharmacokinetic studies showed that pharmacological activity of cilostazol is similar and dose reduction is not required in renally impaired patients [35]. It is unlikely that cilostazol is removed appreciably by dialysis because of its high protein binding.

Previous Antiplatelet Trials in Patients with Hemodialysis

As there have been no randomized controlled trials regarding the optimal antiplatelet agents for secondary prevention of stroke in CKD, knowledge can be extrapolated from previous randomized controlled studies comparing the efficacy and safety of different antiplatelet regimens for prevention of vascular events in hemodialysis patients who had the most severe form of CKD. The study of aspirin plus clopidogrel in patients undergoing hemodialysis who had an established graft was ended early due to an increased risk of bleeding [36]. Moreover, the study failed to demonstrate a benefit of the regimen, as compared with placebo, for the prevention of graft thrombosis.

On the other hand, a recent study showed that treatment with aspirin plus extended-release dipyridamole results in a significant improvement in primary unassisted graft patency compared to placebo [37]. Interestingly, the bleeding risk did not differ between two groups suggesting safety of aspirin plus dipyridamole in these patients (hazard ratio for aspirin plus dipyridamole, 0.86; 95% CI 0.55–1.35). Another trial using propensity score matching investigated the effects of cilostazol administration on long-term patency after percutaneous transluminal angioplasty in hemodialysis patients with peripheral artery disease. The study demonstrated that cilostazol treatment not only prevented restenosis but also reduced mortality including cardiovascular death [38].

Beyond Antiplatelet Therapy

The Study of Heart and Renal Protection (SHARP) trial investigated the efficacy and safety of statin treatment in patients with moderate-to-severe kidney disease and without history of CVD [39]. The trial found a 17% proportional reduction in major atherosclerotic events in the statin-treated group compared with the placebo group, yet no adverse effect on renal function [39]. Furthermore, a recent retrospective observational study showed that statins benefit patients with a history of recent myocardial infarction and stage I–IV CKD [40]. On the contrary, randomized controlled trials of dialysis patients on statin treatment yielded conflicting results [41, 42]. However, patients with atherosclerotic stroke and all stage of CKD should be treated with statins which have been shown both to be safe and well tolerated in patients with CKD just as if their kidney function was normal, because they already had overt atherosclerotic disease [41, 42].

Long-term control of chronic hypertension is the most important factor in stroke prevention, irrespective of the antihypertensive agents used. One distinctive aspect of blood pressure control in those with CKD revealed from epidemiological studies of a J-shaped relationship between blood pressure and stroke [43]. A recent randomized controlled trial, however, clearly demonstrated that a continuous relationship between achieved blood pressure and the risk of recurrent stroke in a CKD population [44]. In patients with DM, angiotensin converting enzyme inhibitors and angiotensin II receptor antagonist are considered as first-line agents in the treatment of hypertension because of their role in preventing and treating diabetic nephropathy. More studies regarding optimal class of antihypertensive drug or target blood pressure level for prevention of stroke in CKD patients are needed.

Table 1. Considerations in prevention of ischemic stroke in chronic kidney disease patients

	Hemorrhagic risk	Platelet inhibition	Endothelial function	Prevent nephropathy
Antiplatelet therapy				
Aspirin	presence	presence	none	possibly harmful
Clopidogrel[1]	presence	presence	none	unknown
Aggrenox	low[3]	presence	beneficial	unknown
Cilostazol[1]	low[3]	presence	beneficial	unknown
Risk factors control				
Antihypertensive agents[2]	beneficial	none	beneficial	beneficial
Statins	controversial	none	beneficial	none

[1] With/without aspirin.
[2] Angiotensin-converting enzyme inhibitors and angiotensin II receptor antagonist.
[3] Compared with aspirin.

Finally, renal transplantation may be the best treatment for solving may clinical problems related to end stage renal disease. The risk of vascular events including cardiac and cerebral complications is lower in transplant recipients compared with transplant candidates awaiting surgery, suggesting cardio- and cerebrovascular-protective benefits of transplantation [45, 46]. In addition, endothelial damage and oxidative stress resulting from renal impairment and uremic toxin are also reduced after renal transplantation [47]. However, the incidence of CVD is 3–4 times higher, even among renal transplant recipients compared with age-matched controls [48]. As underlying vascular risk factors may still be present and possible adverse effects of immunosuppressive agents may exist after transplantation, establishing optimal treatment strategies in these patients is warranted.

Conclusion

CKD may be an independent risk factor of stroke, of which the outcome is poor with a high recurrence rate. Antiplatelet drugs are recommended for reducing stroke risk, especially in patients with non-cardioembolic ischemic stroke. However, specific recommendations for antiplatelet therapy in patients with ischemic stroke plus CKD are not available yet. CKD treatment with a particular antiplatelet agent has to be individualized with several considerations (table 1). Other treatments including lipid management, blood pressure control, and renal transplantation for prevention of stroke in CKD patients are also important. Further studies are warranted for optimal treatment in stroke prevention in CKD patients.

References

1 Roger VL, Go AS, Lloyd-Jones DM, Benjamin EJ, Berry JD, Borden WB, Bravata DM, Dai S, Ford ES, Fox CS, Fullerton HJ, Gillespie C, Hailpern SM, Heit JA, Howard VJ, Kissela BM, Kittner SJ, Lackland DT, Lichtman JH, Lisabeth LD, Makuc DM, Marcus GM, Marelli A, Matchar DB, Moy CS, Mozaffarian D, Mussolino ME, Nichol G, Paynter NP, Soliman EZ, Sorlie PD, Sotoodehnia N, Turan TN, Virani SS, Wong ND, Woo D, Turner MB: Heart disease and stroke statistics – 2012 update: a report from the American Heart Association. Circulation 2012; 125:e2–e220.

2 Go AS, Chertow GM, Fan D, McCulloch CE, Hsu CY: Chronic kidney disease and the risks of death, cardiovascular events, and hospitalization. N Engl J Med 2004;351:1296–1305.

3 Nakayama M, Metoki H, Terawaki H, Ohkubo T, Kikuya M, Sato T, Nakayama K, Asayama K, Inoue R, Hashimoto J, Totsune K, Hoshi H, Ito S, Imai Y: Kidney dysfunction as a risk factor for first symptomatic stroke events in a general Japanese population – the Ohasama study. Nephrol Dial Transplant 2007;22:1910–1915.

4 Wannamethee SG, Shaper AG, Perry IJ: Serum creatinine concentration and risk of cardiovascular disease: a possible marker for increased risk of stroke. Stroke 1997;28: 557–563.

5 Bos MJ, Koudstaal PJ, Hofman A, Breteler MM: Decreased glomerular filtration rate is a risk factor for hemorrhagic but not for ischemic stroke: the Rotterdam Study. Stroke 2007;38:3127–3132.

6 Shimizu Y, Maeda K, Imano H, Ohira T, Kitamura A, Kiyama M, Okada T, Ishikawa Y, Shimamoto T, Yamagishi K, Tanigawa T, Iso H: Chronic kidney disease and drinking status in relation to risks of stroke and its subtypes: the Circulatory Risk in Communities Study (CIRCS). Stroke 2011;42:2531–2537.

7 Kang DH, Kanellis J, Hugo C, Truong L, Anderson S, Kerjaschki D, Schreiner GF, Johnson RJ: Role of the microvascular endothelium in progressive renal disease. J Am Soc Nephrol 2002;13:806–816.

8 Khatri M, Wright CB, Nickolas TL, Yoshita M, Paik MC, Kranwinkel G, Sacco RL, DeCarli C: Chronic kidney disease is associated with white matter hyperintensity volume: the Northern Manhattan Study (NOMAS). Stroke 2007;38:3121–3126.

9 Ikram MA, Vernooij MW, Hofman A, Niessen WJ, van der Lugt A, Breteler MM: Kidney function is related to cerebral small vessel disease. Stroke 2008;39:55–61.

10 Cho AH, Lee SB, Han SJ, Shon YM, Yang DW, Kim BS: Impaired kidney function and cerebral microbleeds in patients with acute ischemic stroke. Neurology 2009;73:1645–1648.

11 Seliger SL, Longstreth WT Jr: Lessons about brain vascular disease from another pulsating organ, the kidney. Stroke 2008;39:5–6.

12 Parfrey PS, Foley RN: The clinical epidemiology of cardiac disease in chronic renal failure. J Am Soc Nephrol 1999;10:1606–1615.

13 MacWalter RS, Wong SY, Wong KY, Stewart G, Fraser CG, Fraser HW, Ersoy Y, Ogston SA, Chen R: Does renal dysfunction predict mortality after acute stroke? A 7-year follow-up study. Stroke 2002;33:1630–1635.

14 Lima HN, Cabral NL, Franklin J, Moro CH, Pecoits-Filho R, Goncalves AR: Age dependent impact of estimated glomerular filtration rate on long-term survival after ischaemic stroke. Nephrology (Carlton) 2012;17: 725–732.

15 Yahalom G, Schwartz R, Schwammenthal Y, Merzeliak O, Toashi M, Orion D, Sela BA, Tanne D: Chronic kidney disease and clinical outcome in patients with acute stroke. Stroke 2009;40:1296–1303.

16 Lyrer PA, Fluri F, Gisler D, Papa S, Hatz F, Engelter ST: Renal function and outcome among stroke patients treated with IV thrombolysis. Neurology 2008;71:1548–1550.

17 Shlipak MG, Heidenreich PA, Noguchi H, Chertow GM, Browner WS, McClellan MB: Association of renal insufficiency with treatment and outcomes after myocardial infarction in elderly patients. Ann Intern Med 2002;137:555–562.

18 Weiner DE, Tighiouart H, Stark PC, Amin MG, MacLeod B, Griffith JL, Salem DN, Levey AS, Sarnak MJ: Kidney disease as a risk factor for recurrent cardiovascular disease and mortality. Am J Kidney Dis 2004;44:198–206.

19 Kuwashiro T, Sugimori H, Ago T, Kamouchi M, Kitazono T: Risk factors predisposing to stroke recurrence within one year of non-cardioembolic stroke onset: the Fukuoka Stroke Registry. Cerebrovasc Dis 2012;33:141–149.
20 Furie KL, Kasner SE, Adams RJ, Albers GW, Bush RL, Fagan SC, Halperin JL, Johnston SC, Katzan I, Kernan WN, Mitchell PH, Ovbiagele B, Palesch YY, Sacco RL, Schwamm LH, Wassertheil-Smoller S, Turan TN, Wentworth D: Guidelines for the prevention of stroke in patients with stroke or transient ischemic attack: a guideline for healthcare professionals from the American Heart Association/American Stroke Association. Stroke 2011;42:227–276.
21 Lansberg MG, O'Donnell MJ, Khatri P, Lang ES, Nguyen-Huynh MN, Schwartz NE, Sonnenberg FA, Schulman S, Vandvik PO, Spencer FA, Alonso-Coello P, Guyatt GH, Akl EA: Antithrombotic and thrombolytic therapy for ischemic stroke: Antithrombotic Therapy and Prevention of Thrombosis, 9th ed: American College of Chest Physicians Evidence-Based Clinical Practice Guidelines. Chest 2012;141:e601S–e636S.
22 Park TH, Kim MK, Oh HG, Oh MS, Yu KH, Hong KS, Bae HJ, Kwon SU, Rha JH, Heo JH, Oh CW, Lee BC, BW Y: Antiplatelet therapy for secondary stroke prevention: 2012 focused update of Korean Clinical Practice Guidelines for Stroke. Korean J Stroke 2012; 14:1–5.
23 Weigert AL, Schafer AI: Uremic bleeding: pathogenesis and therapy. Am J Med Sci 1998;316:94–104.
24 Kaw D, Malhotra D: Platelet dysfunction and end-stage renal disease. Semin Dial 2006;19: 317–322.
25 Jardine MJ, Ninomiya T, Perkovic V, Cass A, Turnbull F, Gallagher MP, Zoungas S, Lambers Heerspink HJ, Chalmers J, Zanchetti A: Aspirin is beneficial in hypertensive patients with chronic kidney disease: a post-hoc subgroup analysis of a randomized controlled trial. J Am Coll Cardiol 2010;56:956–965.
26 Antithrombotic Trialists' Collaboration: Collaborative meta-analysis of randomised trials of antiplatelet therapy for prevention of death, myocardial infarction, and stroke in high risk patients. BMJ 2002;324:71–86.
27 Park SH, Kim W, Park CS, Kang WY, Hwang SH: A comparison of clopidogrel responsiveness in patients with versus without chronic renal failure. Am J Cardiol 2009;104:1292–1295.
28 Mezzano D, Tagle R, Panes O, Perez M, Downey P, Munoz B, Aranda E, Barja P, Thambo S, Gonzalez F, Mezzano S, Pereira J: Hemostatic disorder of uremia: the platelet defect, main determinant of the prolonged bleeding time, is correlated with indices of activation of coagulation and fibrinolysis. Thromb Haemost 1996;76:312–321.
29 Wurtz M, Wulff LN, Grove EL, Kristensen SD, Hvas AM: Influence of renal function and platelet turnover on the antiplatelet effect of aspirin. Thromb Res 2012;129:434–440.
30 Angiolillo DJ, Bernardo E, Capodanno D, Vivas D, Sabate M, Ferreiro JL, Ueno M, Jimenez-Quevedo P, Alfonso F, Bass TA, Macaya C, Fernandez-Ortiz A: Impact of chronic kidney disease on platelet function profiles in diabetes mellitus patients with coronary artery disease taking dual antiplatelet therapy. J Am Coll Cardiol 2010;55:1139–1146.
31 Woo JS, Kim W, Lee SR, Jung KH, Kim WS, Lew JH, Lee TW, Lim CK: Platelet reactivity in patients with chronic kidney disease receiving adjunctive cilostazol compared with a high-maintenance dose of clopidogrel: results of the effect of platelet inhibition according to clopidogrel dose in patients with chronic kidney disease (PIANO-2 CKD) randomized study. Am Heart J 2011;162:1018–1025.
32 Shinohara Y, Katayama Y, Uchiyama S, Yamaguchi T, Handa S, Matsuoka K, Ohashi Y, Tanahashi N, Yamamoto H, Genka C, Kitagawa Y, Kusuoka H, Nishimaru K, Tsushima M, Koretsune Y, Sawada T, Hamada C: Cilostazol for prevention of secondary stroke (CSPS 2): an aspirin-controlled, double-blind, randomised non-inferiority trial. Lancet Neurol 2010;9:959–968.
33 Trovati M, Cavalot F: Optimization of hypolipidemic and antiplatelet treatment in the diabetic patient with renal disease. J Am Soc Nephrol 2004;15(suppl 1):S12–S20.
34 Fored CM, Ejerblad E, Lindblad P, Fryzek JP, Dickman PW, Signorello LB, Lipworth L, Elinder CG, Blot WJ, McLaughlin JK, Zack MM, Nyren O: Acetaminophen, aspirin, and chronic renal failure. N Engl J Med 2001;345: 1801–1808.

35 Mallikaarjun S, Forbes WP, Bramer SL: Effect of renal impairment on the pharmacokinetics of cilostazol and its metabolites. Clin Pharmacokinet 1999;37(suppl 2):33–40.
36 Kaufman JS, O'Connor TZ, Zhang JH, Cronin RE, Fiore LD, Ganz MB, Goldfarb DS, Peduzzi PN: Randomized controlled trial of clopidogrel plus aspirin to prevent hemodialysis access graft thrombosis. J Am Soc Nephrol 2003;14:2313–2321.
37 Dixon BS, Beck GJ, Vazquez MA, Greenberg A, Delmez JA, Allon M, Dember LM, Himmelfarb J, Gassman JJ, Greene T, Radeva MK, Davidson IJ, Ikizler TA, Braden GL, Fenves AZ, Kaufman JS, Cotton JR Jr, Martin KJ, McNeil JW, Rahman A, Lawson JH, Whiting JF, Hu B, Meyers CM, Kusek JW, Feldman HI: Effect of dipyridamole plus aspirin on hemodialysis graft patency. N Engl J Med 2009;360:2191–2201.
38 Ishii H, Kumada Y, Toriyama T, Aoyama T, Takahashi H, Yamada S, Yasuda Y, Yuzawa Y, Maruyama S, Matsuo S, Matsubara T, Murohara T: Cilostazol improves long-term patency after percutaneous transluminal angioplasty in hemodialysis patients with peripheral artery disease. Clin J Am Soc Nephrol 2008;3:1034–1040.
39 Baigent C, Landray MJ, Reith C, Emberson J, Wheeler DC, Tomson C, Wanner C, Krane V, Cass A, Craig J, Neal B, Jiang L, Hooi LS, Levin A, Agodoa L, Gaziano M, Kasiske B, Walker R, Massy ZA, Feldt-Rasmussen B, Krairittichai U, Ophascharoensuk V, Fellstrom B, Holdaas H, Tesar V, Wiecek A, Grobbee D, de Zeeuw D, Gronhagen-Riska C, Dasgupta T, Lewis D, Herrington W, Mafham M, Majoni W, Wallendszus K, Grimm R, Pedersen T, Tobert J, Armitage J, Baxter A, Bray C, Chen Y, Chen Z, Hill M, Knott C, Parish S, Simpson D, Sleight P, Young A, Collins R: The effects of lowering LDL cholesterol with simvastatin plus ezetimibe in patients with chronic kidney disease (Study of Heart and Renal Protection): a randomised placebo-controlled trial. Lancet 2011;377:2181–2192.
40 Szummer K, Lundman P, Jacobson SH, Schon S, Lindback J, Stenestrand U, Wallentin L, Jernberg T: Association between statin treatment and outcome in relation to renal function in survivors of myocardial infarction. Kidney Int 2011;79:997–1004.
41 Jenkins M, Goldsmith D: Statins and kidney disease: is the study of heart and renal protection at the cutting edge of evidence? Curr Opin Cardiol 2012;27:429–440.
42 Heymann EP, Kassimatis TI, Goldsmith DJ: Dyslipidemia, statins, and CKD patients' outcomes – review of the evidence in the post-sharp era. J Nephrol 2012;25:460–472.
43 Weiner DE, Tighiouart H, Levey AS, Elsayed E, Griffith JL, Salem DN, Sarnak MJ: Lowest systolic blood pressure is associated with stroke in stages 3 to 4 chronic kidney disease. J Am Soc Nephrol 2007;18:960–966.
44 Ninomiya T, Perkovic V, Gallagher M, Jardine M, Cass A, Arima H, Anderson C, Neal B, Woodward M, Omae T, MacMahon S, Chalmers J: Lower blood pressure and risk of recurrent stroke in patients with chronic kidney disease: PROGRESS trial. Kidney Int 2008;73:963–970.
45 Meier-Kriesche HU, Schold JD, Srinivas TR, Reed A, Kaplan B: Kidney transplantation halts cardiovascular disease progression in patients with end-stage renal disease. Am J Transplant 2004;4:1662–1668.
46 Lentine KL, Rocca Rey LA, Kolli S, Bacchi G, Schnitzler MA, Abbott KC, Xiao H, Brennan DC: Variations in the risk for cerebrovascular events after kidney transplant compared with experience on the waiting list and after graft failure. Clin J Am Soc Nephrol 2008;3:1090–1101.
47 Kocak H, Ceken K, Yavuz A, Yucel S, Gurkan A, Erdogan O, Ersoy F, Yakupoglu G, Demirbas A, Tuncer M: Effect of renal transplantation on endothelial function in haemodialysis patients. Nephrol Dial Transplant 2006;21:203–207.
48 Kasiske BL: Risk factors for accelerated atherosclerosis in renal transplant recipients. Am J Med 1988;84:985–992.

Oh Young Bang, MD, PhD
Department of Neurology and the Stroke and Cerebrovascular Center
Samsung Medical Center, Sungkyunkwan University
50 Irwon-dong, Gangnam-gu, Seoul 135-710 (South Korea)
E-Mail nmboy@unitel.co.kr

Author Index

Subject Index